PRAISE
RESTORE YOUR LIFE FROM CHRONIC PAIN

"If you suffer from chronic pain, you want a way out that is practical—and one that works. This book describes an elegant and powerful program that achieves both. Dr. Weisberg is a master guide who has led many others back to health. Let him show you how to restore your own life from the throes of chronic pain."

—**Henry Emmons, MD**, author of *The Chemistry of Joy and The Chemistry of Calm*

"Dr. Weisberg has culled his extensive interdisciplinary and integrative medicine experience assisting patients with chronic pain move to a fuller, comfortable life into this groundbreaking guide for personal recovery. In *Restore Your Life from Chronic Pain*, he masterfully explains the impact of pain, the role of neuroplasticity in its development, and translates the latest neuroscience into strategies anyone can use to modify their pain experience permanently. His ABC model of the self-healing journey is beautifully illustrated and captures the wisdom he has accrued from helping countless people recover. Not only will this book educate and guide you to a comfortable and satisfying life, but it will also equip clinicians from all disciplines with the skills to help their patients return to a life worth living. This is an essential resource for patients and professionals alike."

—**Louis F. Damis, PhD, ABPP**, clinical health psychologist, assistant professor of psychology at the University of Central Florida College of Medicine, and president of the American Society of Clinical Hypnosis

"I have witnessed first-hand how Dr. Weisberg helps people who had failed to respond to many and all prior pain treatments. His new book, *Restore Your Life from Chronic Pain*, shares his gift and wisdom for patients and future generations of health care professionals. A must read for everyone, as pain touches all our lives. This book will restore realistic hope and create meaningful change in people with chronic pain."

—**Alfred L. Clavel Jr., MD**, neurologist, pain Specialist, and former department chair of pain medicine for Health Partners Health Systems

"When patients suffer from chronic pain, they need to understand what has happened to them, and they need effective, usable strategies to help them feel better now. Dr. Weisberg's book, *Restore Your Life from Chronic Pain*, provides comprehensive and powerful ways to rise above and conquer the suffering. His ABC Method provides tangible, time-tested strategies to bring dependable relief. This is an invaluable guide for patients, families, and clinicians as well. A must-read for anyone suffering from chronic pain."

—**Steven Gurgevich, PhD**, former director of the Mind-Body Clinic and clinical assistant professor of medicine at the Andrew Weil Center for Integrative Medicine at the University of Arizona College of Medicine

RESTORE YOUR LIFE FROM CHRONIC PAIN

RESTORE YOUR LIFE FROM CHRONIC PAIN

Find Lasting Relief
from Arthritis, Headache,
and Back Pain

MARK B. WEISBERG, PHD, ABPP

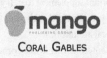

CORAL GABLES

Cover & Layout Design: Megan Werner
Cover Photo: Alex / stock.adobe.com
Interior graphics: leremy, photoplotnikov, pikovit / stock.adobe.com
Illustrator: Jenny Fine

For permission requests, please contact the publisher at:
Mango Publishing Group
2850 S Douglas Road, 2nd Floor
Coral Gables, FL 33134 USA
info@mango.bz

For special orders, quantity sales, course adoptions and corporate sales, please email the publisher at sales@mango.bz. For trade and wholesale sales, please contact Ingram Publisher Services at customer.service@ingramcontent.com or +1.800.509.4887.

Restore Your Life from Chronic Pain: Find Lasting Relief from Arthritis, Headache, and Back Pain

Library of Congress Cataloging-in-Publication number: 2023943738
ISBN: (pb) 978-1-68481-422-0 (hc) 978-1-68481-423-7
(e) 978-1-68481-424-4
BISAC category code: HEA036000 HEALTH & FITNESS / Pain Management

Disclaimer

The information provided in this book is not intended as a substitute for professional medical advice, but as an important supplement to it. If you are experiencing any serious symptoms that you have not yet discussed with your physician or other health care professional, please seek medical attention.

The patient stories presented in this book come from many years of clinical experience. To protect privacy, all identifying characteristics and data have been changed.

Table of Contents

THE ABC METHOD AWARENESS, BALANCING, AND CULTIVATING

Introduction

WHY I WROTE THIS BOOK

I wrote this book for you.

Chronic pain has taken over your life and is holding you captive. Its grip can last for years, no matter how many new kinds of medications and treatments you try, no matter how many specialists you see. Often you find temporary relief, but when the pain returns, you become increasingly frustrated and hopeless. You never feel quite well enough to do the things you used to do, and there seems to be no path forward.

It is for you—a person with chronic pain who wants a normal life—that I am writing this book. I want you to know that there is a way out. There is a way to reclaim your body's natural capacity to heal and recover. To return to the activities of daily life that are meaningful and important to you.

In other words, to *restore your life*.

Over the last thirty-six years, I have seen countless people—just like you—who find their way out of this suffering and return to their normal lives. The secret to this success is a more comprehensive approach to treating chronic pain, one that integrates the newest scientific findings in psychology, medicine, and neuroscience. I was fortunate to begin my career as a clinical health psychologist in 1984, at a pain clinic devoted to integrative medicine. It is clearly the wave of the future. Our treatments for chronic pain are so effective that we attract patients from neighboring states.

The strength of this holistic treatment is not another medicine or implant, but rather the most powerful healing agent known to modern science: the self-healing powers of the human being. In this book I will explain how you can activate your innate self-healing resources and reclaim your life from the grip of chronic pain.

YOUR SELF-HEALING POWER

We possess the natural capacity for restoration.

Self-healing capacities are constantly at work in your body, even down to the cellular level. You may not have thought about it, but your cells are constantly at work healing themselves when they are damaged and replacing themselves with newer, healthier cells. For example, when you fracture a bone, almost immediately your body produces new bone cells to repair the break. When you scrape your knee, the blood clots to stop any bleeding, your immune system activates white blood cells to remove the injured cells, and newer, healthy cells replace the damaged skin. Our body is in a constant state of repairing damage and producing healthier tissue.

Statistically, up to 90 percent of all illnesses and other health problems resolve without medical intervention. Think of all the times you, your spouse, or your child had a stomachache, sore throat, headache, or common cold that got better without going to a hospital or primary care clinic.

SELF-CARE AND GENETICS

Striving to understand the mystery of how mind-body healing occurs is what drives my career and is the ultimate inspiration for this book. My quest eventually led me to explore the role of genetics in the healing process.

Genetics are an important contributing factor in your health. Your genes determine, for example, that you may be five foot, eight inches tall with green eyes, or that you have a vulnerability to joint soreness, dry skin, or muscle aches. Unfortunately, some people are born with a genetic loading for higher pain sensitivity than the general population. They feel pain more intensely than most people.

However, your genetic predisposition is only part of the story. Take for example stomach ulcers, long considered to be one of the "classic seven psychosomatic disorders." Then, in 1982, researchers found a link between ulcers and the *H. pylori* bacteria. This changed the common wisdom about ulcers, and soon they were treated with antibiotics—not psychotherapy.

As years passed, researchers discovered an interesting anomaly: Not everyone who had the gene for *H. pylori* ulcers developed stomach ulcers! This meant that some nongenetic factor played a role in who developed ulcers. They found that the people who had genetic vulnerability to H. pylori ulcers but didn't get ulcers tended to practice healthy habits—eating a balanced diet, getting sufficient sleep, practicing stress management techniques, addressing difficult emotional stressors, etc.

We now know that chronic health conditions such as stomach ulcers are caused by multiple factors. It is not a rigid either/or. They are not strictly caused only by either emotional stressors or genetics. Rather, stomach ulcers arise from a combination of factors, including *H. pylori* bacteria, acid reflux, frequent use of certain pain medications such as ibuprofen, frequent use of steroid medications, and unresolved emotional stresses. Emotional stresses in isolation alone usually aren't enough to cause ulcers, but they can certainly contribute to the development of ulcers. Unresolved emotional stresses can affect the immune system as well as brain–gut communication, and that combination can make the difference in who gets ulcers.

These insights relate to the field of scientific research known as *epigenetics*, how your behavior and environment can activate or suppress certain genes. I learned from epigenetics how positive self–care activities can beneficially affect our health even when we possess genes for various kinds of diseases. Epigenetics taught me that the ways we take care of our stresses, our diet, and our needs for rest and exercise, play a crucial role in how we heal from chronic pain.

THE STORY OF JANICE—
A CHRONIC PAIN SUFFERER

Here is a story that may sound familiar to you. I have heard variations of it from hundreds of patients. It is the story of Janice, a virtual composite of many patients I have treated.

Janice, a forty-eight-year-old mother of two, had chronic back pain for five years. She worked as a paralegal for a big law firm downtown. Her back pain began with a single mishap. She was on her way to a church and had to bring a box of items she was donating to a rummage sale for an African mission. She had lifted up a heavy box about a foot off the floor when she felt a sharp pain in her lower back, like being struck by a bolt of lightning. "I screamed so loud that my ten-year-old and eight-year-old came running to see what was wrong," Janice said.

She went to her internist, Dr. Stevens, who initially gave her ibuprofen and stretching exercises to do. When that didn't work, Janice saw an orthopedic surgeon who found a herniated disc and operated on it.

"That seemed to help quite a bit at first, along with the physical therapy," Janice said. "But it was really difficult to find time to do the exercises and go to all the appointments because I was so busy with my boys and work and everything else. I did the best I could because so many people depend on me. After all that, the pain never really went away, so I was miserable and frustrated at the same time."

After a couple of years of lingering pain, she started thinking the surgery hadn't worked. Her entire low back was stiff and sore, and she would get jolts of pain shooting down her right leg, all the way down to her foot. She figured she needed another surgery, so she returned to the orthopedist. He did an MRI and said it looked fine. The surgery was successful, and the disc was healed. As such, there was nothing more he could do.

"I went to a different orthopedic surgeon for a second opinion but was told the same thing. My disc was okay, so that was that."

Janice then sought out several other specialists, hoping to find some help. She went to a neurologist who ordered nerve conduction tests and prescribed an anticonvulsant medication for her pain—gabapentin. It worked a little bit, but it made her drowsy and she started gaining weight. Then she went to a physiatrist, who specializes in physical medicine and rehabilitation. He injected steroids into her lower back. After each of the four shots she felt better for a while, but then the pain and stiffness came back full force.

Subsequently she consulted with another neurologist, a rheumatologist, two other physical therapists, a craniosacral therapist, an acupuncturist, and a chiropractor. All of that provided little if any relief. By this time she was also taking several prescription drugs: a narcotic pain pill, a muscle relaxant, an antidepressant to help nerve pain, a tranquilizer, and two different medications for sleep.

After five years of seeking various treatments that didn't work, Janice returned to her internist, Dr. Stevens. She told Janice that all the diagnostic tests were negative. "That means that your symptoms are not due to something serious like cancer or degenerative neurological disease." She then discussed lifestyle changes and stress reduction. Dr. Stevens also mentioned that Janice might benefit from seeing a psychologist to address some of the stresses affecting her symptoms. Now Janice was feeling demoralized— "Does Dr. Stevens think the problem is all in my head?"

The psychologist evaluated Janice for depression and anxiety, thinking that the pain might be due to repressed emotional problems. He told Janice, "I don't think you have psychological problems significant enough to warrant treatment, so I don't think my services would be helpful to you at this time."

After all the consultations and treatments, Janice lost hope for relief. "I feel like there's nowhere else to turn."

Janice's frustration is shared by a majority of health professionals who see patients like Janice but have limited impact on solving their problems. Despite the diligent and caring work of these clinicians, Janice and millions of others find only limited relief for their chronic pain. What Janice didn't realize was that she wasn't alone in her frustration and hopelessness.

"WHAT ELSE CAN BE DONE?"

All these patients share the same story of a fruitless search for a way to rid themselves of chronic pain, though their specific ailments may differ. I have worked with patients with a wide range of conditions, everything from chronic headache to low back pain, fibromyalgia, TMJ and chronic facial pain, neuropathic pain (like trigeminal neuralgia), cancer pain, IBS and chronic abdominal pain, chronic fatigue syndrome, and complex regional pain syndrome (CRPS, formerly known as reflex sympathetic dystrophy)—just to name a few.

By the time these patients are referred to me, their big question is, "What else can be done?"

My job is to gain a holistic understanding of my patients' problems—keeping in mind the ways the body and mind work together—and then guide them as they discover and activate their inner self-healing resources. Over the years of providing direct patient care, I noticed that certain practices, exercises, and skills reliably activated their self-healing properties. While each case is unique in its own way, it became apparent that a common set of factors must be addressed to improve stubborn chronic pain symptoms and help create long-lasting relief. I learned more about these factors in many ways—ongoing case review with my colleagues, teaching at pain medicine conferences, and supervising residents and interns. The pattern of effective practices that emerged made the complex problem of chronic pain simpler, and it formed the basis of the guided program of self-healing that I present in this book.

THE ABC METHOD FOR
HEALING CHRONIC PAIN

The way to reduce chronic pain by activating your self-healing powers is captured in the acronym ABC, which stands for Awareness, Balancing, and Cultivating. The ABC method will teach you new ways to deal with your chronic pain and empower you to break free from the vicious cycle of distress, fear, frustration, and despair.

AWARENESS

Activating your internal healing abilities starts with awareness. First of all, you need to pay attention to the sensations of your body, because this is your body's way of trying to tell you something. Its wisdom is lost if you don't listen to it. Focusing your awareness sounds easy, but it can be quite tricky and elusive. That's because we all have a natural tendency to avoid things that feel painful, and many chronic pain sufferers ignore their pain habitually. They mask it with medications, or distract themselves with mindless activities or social media to divert their awareness from bodily sensations.

The art of awareness entails learning effective strategies to become aware of your emotions and thoughts, as well as your physical sensations. Only then can you tune in to your body's natural capacity to change and heal. Awareness is a prerequisite for the skills that follow.

How do you describe your pain?

- Burning
- Tight
- Throbbing
- Aching

- Tingling
- Stiff
- Shooting
- Stinging

BALANCING

Balance has been a central concept in medicine and healing for centuries. The idea is that we are complex creatures with multiple processes going on at the same time. These functions need to be balanced for us to be healthy. The goal is to achieve equilibrium. Our nervous system maintains a balance between its energizing influence and its calming influence. When we move, some muscles contract while others lengthen and relax. Our immune system does a constant balancing act between activating cells that attack germs and cells that quiet down the attack. Every day our lives seek a balance between activity and rest or social interaction and solitude. And we all know we need a balanced diet.

From an integrative medicine perspective, health and healing result from establishing balance on multiple levels. The art of balancing involves learning various ways to support your mind and body with that much-needed equilibrium.

CULTIVATING

Activating your self-healing powers—your capacity for restoration—doesn't happen by itself, a lesson we learned from epigenetics. Sustained pain relief requires cultivating new habits. This ongoing effort to activate your self-healing resources leads you to the rewards you seek—restoration, resilience, and healing. We possess the potential for these kinds of positive changes, and cultivating proper self-care habits will trigger the most powerful pain-relieving systems in the body. The "Cultivating" section of the book will tell you how to do exactly that.

A key component of cultivation is the notion of a resource tank, your reservoir of skills, strategies, and energy that ensure quicker healing. You will learn how to keep your resource tank full by acquiring such special skills as self-hypnosis and Limbic Retraining—a technique that uses your mind to calm your brain.

The ABC guided program to reduce chronic pain is an entirely different approach than the quick fix of medications, trigger point injections, and implantable pain pumps. True primary care is not what your physician does for you, but rather what you do for yourself. You are in the driver's seat, and this book will guide you on your journey.

ARE YOU READY TO USE THIS BOOK?

I cannot help you address your chronic pain unless you have first had medical evaluation for any physical problems you might have. A prerequisite for starting the ABC journey is that you have a physical diagnosis for your pain. That means you must be evaluated by a primary care physician or a physician pain specialist who rules out any serious or life-threatening problems. Any conditions and symptoms that might be associated with a more serious illness should be comprehensively tested and treated. Otherwise, you are not ready for this book.

Once you have been medically evaluated and organic conditions have been addressed, yet your pain continues for at least three to six months, you are ready for this book.

If your health care provider diagnoses your chronic pain as one of these conditions, there is no doubt that you qualify to begin the ABC healing journey:

- Arthritis or joint pain (either osteoarthritis or rheumatoid arthritis)

- Back pain

- Neck pain

- Cancer pain

- Headaches, including migraine and daily tension headache

- Persisting pain in scar tissue

- Muscle pain all over (such as with fibromyalgia)

- Chronic pelvic pain (including interstitial cystitis)

- Jaw pain/facial pain/temporomandibular pain (TMD)

- Peripheral neuropathy (tingling and burning caused by damage to nerves, primarily in your hands and feet)

- Chronic digestive pain, such as IBS, gastritis or GERD

- Myofascial pain syndrome

- Herniated lumbar disc

- Lyme disease

- Endometriosis

The good news is that these frustrating conditions are not life-threatening. The problem for chronic pain sufferers is not that they will die from it, but that it becomes increasingly difficult to live with it.

Most chronic pain sufferers—like Janice—continue to search for possible physiological causes of their pain, even after the original injury has healed. When the primary care physician can no longer find any physical illness or disease process that might be responsible for generating the pain, people like Janice continue their search by seeing all kinds of specialists. They may spend years running the gauntlet of orthopedists, neurologists, physical medicine and rehabilitation specialists, psychologists, physical therapists, chiropractors, psychiatrists, acupuncturists, massage therapists, and even nutritionists. Each new specialist provides hope, and quite possibly temporary relief, but the suffering continues and gradually gets worse. Instead of finding their way back to their normal life, people get bogged down in the quagmire of dead ends, detours, and disappointments.

It is common for chronic pain patients to check out various kinds of treatments: numerous medications and supplements, trigger point injections, Botox, physical therapy stretches, ultrasound, intrathecal drug implants or spinal cord stimulators, TENS units, and more. Once again, they find limited relief at best. The longer they go without finding lasting relief for their suffering, the more likely they are to feel exhausted, confused, and discouraged.

If you have suffered for months and years with chronic pain, you are all too familiar with this dreary, never-ending scenario. On one hand, you are trying to live your life while coping with chronic pain. At the same time, you are intent on finding relief, so you travel a treacherous path, struggling to stay on a winding and rocky trail that leads to nowhere.

From my perspective as a proponent of integrative medicine, the answer is obvious. These patients are lost because they are looking for solutions in the wrong place. They are seeking old solutions to new problems. Instead, they need to look in another place: the multidisciplinary territory of integrative medicine, which treats chronic pain from multiple perspectives—physically, psychologically, socially. We understand that chronic pain may have different causes than your original pain, even though they might feel the same.

In the case of chronic pain, a slipped disc or swollen joints alone do not completely explain why your pain persists. Otherwise, the treatments that you have already received would have been more helpful or provided longer-lasting relief. You need to change direction and find better treatments, but you need some help to do it.

What you need is a map that clarifies your situation and shows you how to go from a place of suffering and hopelessness back to your normal life. You are traveling from the traditional idea of physical pain and into the new territory of chronic pain. The two have many differences, and that means the treatments must differ as well. This map will highlight an important area that may be new to you—an inside look at how the body, mind, and emotions interact at the neurological level to affect the intensity and duration of chronic pain. This information is important to have before you undertake the ABC journey to self-healing from chronic pain.

You will also need a guide to show you the route, and the means to deal with any obstacles. You will need trail signs along the way, to help you stay on the path when you occasionally lose your way. As you become reoriented to your new direction, your sense of hope will grow as you realize that you have at last found a way out.

HOW TO USE THIS BOOK

This book is essentially a travel guide for your journey of self-healing. I have guided chronic pain patients on healing journeys over this terrain for over thirty-six years. I have discovered where the dead ends are. I know where the roadblocks and obstacles are hidden. Such guidance will enable you to find your path to healing and stay on it until you find your way back to your regular life with greatly reduced pain and suffering.

You must make certain preparations before you begin. You need the proper resources and training, just as you would for any challenging expedition. The first two parts of the book are devoted to preparing you for your journey by providing an orientation on chronic pain and pinpointing your starting place. The final three parts of the book are devoted to the three types of self-care activities in the ABC program that will move you along the path: Awareness, Balance, and Cultivation.

PART ONE—THE NATURE OF CHRONIC PAIN

The first thing you need is a map to give you some background about the nature of chronic pain and its treatment. This vital first step in your healing process will give you an understanding of the nature of chronic pain—its causes, its complications, and its treatments. We will delve into the neuroscience of chronic pain and show how it is intrinsically connected to your brain, your thoughts, your memories, and your emotions.

You will learn about the important differences between chronic pain and acute (short-lived) pain. You will find out how the nervous system can be damaged and distorted by chronic pain, and what is needed to help it recover. Also, many chronic pain sufferers are frustrated because the medications they take for their ongoing distress don't work very well, even though they are more often effective for acute pain. A chapter in this section provides welcome clarification on this perplexing issue. All of this knowledge about how chronic pain affects your body will explain why you can be hopeful about reducing your pain and suffering.

PART TWO—SETTING THE STAGE

There are several things you must do to be ready to start on a new healing path. At the top of the agenda is to pinpoint your starting place. To get your bearings, we need to look at the map and figure out where to put the little star that says, "You are Here." The way we do this is by having you fill out a Personal Pain Assessment, just like you would if you were meeting with me at my pain clinic. It will help identify where you are on your healing journey.

You will not be making this journey alone. Your guides on this journey will be your healing team, which I will help you to assemble. It typically includes a primary care physician, a clinical psychologist, and a physical therapist.

However, you will be behind the wheel on this trip. Unlike your previous treatments, in which you were a passive recipient of a medication or medical procedure, the path to healing from chronic pain requires you to provide your own treatment—this is a path of self-care. You alone have the ability to carry out the activities and practices that will activate your self-healing potential.

Another part of the challenge of chronic pain is the uncertainty and unpredictability that are part of the process. In the chapter entitled "Your Healing Map," you will find a valuable guide to the trajectory of recovering from chronic pain, with powerful tools for managing the inevitable ups and downs of the healing process.

Once you have gone through these initial steps, you are ready to learn and practice the ABC method for healing chronic pain—Awareness, Balance, and Cultivation.

PART THREE—AWARENESS

We have already mentioned that you need to train yourself to explicitly pay attention to your bodily sensations, your emotions, and your thoughts. This self-monitoring is essential to know where you are and where you are going. It will be a challenge for many of you to break the habit of ignoring your pain and trying to dissociate from it. Specific aspects of your life also call for greater awareness, like paying attention to your stress, your quality of sleep, and your diet.

PART FOUR—BALANCING

Finding balance is both an orientation and an activity. Each of us is a complex system, where all the parts and functions are interconnected. Imbalance furthers chronic pain, whereas balance is needed for healing to occur. In this section you will learn techniques to promote balance of your state of mind and body through grounding exercises and breathing exercises. Other areas that require balance include pacing (not too fast and not too slow), alone time versus social time, and physical balance in terms of posture and strength.

PART FIVE—CULTIVATING

This section emphasizes the special tools and skills you will need to have a successful healing journey. I introduce the notion of a resource tank, which you can replenish to sustain your momentum. The unique method of Limbic Retraining will enable you to calm down your brain's overactive alarm system. Clinical hypnosis can address the overactive components of your brain's pain network. There are a number of ways you can deal with difficult emotions—especially repressed emotions—by recognizing them and processing them. The important contribution of physical exercise helps to energize and support the entire effort. Finally, you will gain important skills for successfully dealing with a pain flare episode, so you can stay on track with your healing.

BENEFITS YOU WILL GAIN FROM THE ABC METHOD

My goal for you is to develop your own personal resource tank of strategies and skills to heal your chronic pain and live a better life. By embracing and using the ABC method, you will be able to achieve the following outcomes:

- Reduce the intensity and frequency of pain

- Reduce the intrusiveness of pain in daily life

- Reduce the hypersensitivity of your central nervous system

- Correct the imbalance of your autonomic nervous system and have a more regulated response to stress

- Heal your communication gap with the sensations of your body—be less afraid of them and more attentive, more able to treat sensations as valuable information from your body about what it needs to feel well

- Gain accurate information about chronic pain, how it progresses, and how it manifests in your body

- Be able to accurately evaluate your pain intensity, frequency, and intrusiveness

- Have an improved sense of your body mechanics, and what it feels like to hold your body in proper postural position

- Reduce reactivity and agitation in response to your pain sensations

- Participate in life optimally, enjoy life more fully, and return to normal engagement in your day-to-day activities

- Increasing sense of emotional well-being

- Increase your physical activity to optimal levels

- Improve sleep and reduce fatigue

Now that I have previewed the ABC method for you, let's get back and see what happened to Janice with low back pain as her treatment with me progressed:

At each appointment, I helped Janice to become aware of ways that she guarded and braced her muscles—because sometimes it was so subtle that she wouldn't have noticed it otherwise. As her rehabilitation progressed, I prompted Janice to engage her somatic awareness to notice the sometimes-small improvements in symptoms from week to week. Each step forward provided tangible evidence of realistic hope to counteract the hopelessness that is so commonplace in chronic pain patients.

After two months, Janice rated the intensity of pain at 3, down from her original assessment of 7. The intrusiveness of her pain dropped from 8 to 2. She was very heartened by these results.

"For the first time since my life of pain began, I feel like I have my hands untied from behind my back. I have better sleep because it's less disrupted by pain, and I am starting to be more engaged in my work and with my family and friends. I have more energy to pay proper attention to my sons. They've even commented on how happy I look. When I do have a flare-up of back pain, I'm not so freaked out by it because I know I'm getting better at learning how to calm down my nervous system and feel more balanced."

Janice came in for two more appointments. Her pain decreased even more, letting her return more fully back into her daily life. She was able to phase out her sleep medications and two pain medications. She had followed the ABC formula to a T. She first gained Awareness of the unique dynamics of chronic pain, and learned to pay a different kind of attention to her bodily sensations, emotions, and trigger. She practiced calming techniques and stress management strategies to Balance her body/mind systems. And she committed herself to Cultivate self-healing capacities within herself through regular practice of rejuvenating skills.

Treatment was successful and was ended. She promised me—and herself—that she would keep up her new healthy habits and enjoy her life again.

I wish you well on your healing journey. I am confident that the techniques and skills you learn from this book will significantly reduce your suffering and increase your feelings of well-being and vitality.

Mark Weisberg, PhD, ABPP
Summer, 2023

SECTION I

The Science
of Chronic Pain

CHAPTER 1

What Is Pain?

Each of us has an intimate familiarity with pain. We may not be able to define it, but we know it when we feel it. This personal consciousness of pain is the key indicator of your problem, which is why the ABC method for healing chronic pain begins with awareness.

The unpleasant feeling of pain is a purely subjective experience. No one else has access to that feeling but you. Only you can rate its intensity on a scale of zero to ten. Only you can tell the doctor whether the pain is aching, stabbing, or dull. Only you can point to where it hurts.

Pain has a way of demanding your attention. A sudden jolt of pain can grab your mind instantly, while all other concerns are suspended. At other times, pain is a mere nuisance—like when you have a faint temporary stomachache. And then there is chronic pain—a bothersome pain that just won't go away. The lingering pain becomes part of your environment, an unwelcome presence that takes over and dominates your life. This is what happens in all varieties of chronic pain—like debilitating chronic low back pain, migraine headaches, or fibromyalgia.

There is no mistaking the presence of pain.

People who study pain for a living have come up with an objective definition of pain: "An unpleasant sensory and emotional experience associated with actual or potential tissue damage" (International Association for the Study of Pain (IASP)).

This definition has three components. You already understand the first part, that pain is an unpleasant sensory experience. This includes all the various sorts of pain—sharp, dull, stabbing, aching, and so on.

Pain creates a second mode of experience, and that is the feeling of emotions. Mixed in with the sensory awareness of pain are all kinds of emotions (feelings)—irritation, frustration, depression, despair, heaviness, agitation, or upset. People tend to think of emotions as something experienced in their heads, but if you tune into these feelings, you will notice that you can feel them only through your body, and nowhere else. Excitement manifests as butterflies in the stomach, depression comes across as a heavy, hollow feeling in the chest, fear as a tightness in the forehead and a racing heart. (The next time you feel emotional, try to notice *where* it is in your body.)

The entanglement of pain and emotion is no surprise from the perspective of neuroscience. That's because the brain's "pain network" literally overlaps with the brain's "emotion network." The same areas are activated, the same bundles of neurons. This link provides us with a strong clue for how to treat chronic pain. As you learn more about how pain and emotion interact, you'll discover how this awareness can empower you.

The third component of the IASP definition of pain is that it is associated with "actual or potential tissue damage." This refers to the function of painful sensations as warning signals to notify you of damage to your body. The purpose of ordinary pain is to let us know that something is wrong. If you trip while running and your ankle hurts, the pain prompts you to rest it, ice it, or perhaps go to a physician and have it checked out.

Clinicians cannot measure pain objectively, because only *you* can feel it. But they can search for its origin and determine the severity of any injuries by conducting various examinations and tests. Their methods of investigation include physical examinations, X-rays, CT scans, MRIs, blood tests, and other tools. If you experience a sharp stabbing pain in your lower right abdomen, for example, clinicians will check for appendicitis, among various possible causes. They may track the source of your various pain symptoms to a broken bone, a ruptured disc, an undetected tumor, or other undiagnosed illness.

Pain is more than just an unpleasant sensation, because it also conveys meaning. Pain carries the message that something is wrong and you need to deal with it. Each flash of pain is supposed to be a warning signal about actual or potential danger. The thoughts we have about our pain (such as "This will pass quickly" or "This pain is sucking all the joy out of my life") greatly affect the intensity of our suffering. Pain and its perceived meaning play an essential role in protecting your health.

The Nature of Pain

The International Association for the Study of Pain (IASP) provides a clinical definition of pain: "An unpleasant sensory and emotional experience associated with actual or potential tissue damage."

- Pain is a subjective feeling
  - Pain cannot be objectively measured
- Pain is a sensation intermingled with emotion
  - The brain network that processes pain overlaps with the network that processes emotion
- Pain normally functions as a symptom of something wrong
  - Pain typically indicates actual or potential bodily damage

---

THE DANGER OF NOT FEELING PAIN

If you absent-mindedly put your hand on a hot stove, the sharp pain in your fingers alerts you to potential harm, and you reflexively pull your hand away from the stove before it gets seriously burned.

We need to be able to feel pain to survive and be well. In fact, people who can't feel acute pain are in danger of serious injury. Several years ago a colleague of mine, Dr. Mike Taylor, was invited to visit a hospital in India. He was there to see their outpatient program for people with leprosy, a disease that can interfere with the body's nerve signals. Dr. Taylor went on rounds, attended lectures, and learned from specialists who were at the forefront of treating leprosy. At a social gathering that included patients with leprosy, someone asked him to open a jar of canned fruit that they couldn't get open. He gave it a try, but couldn't do it because the lid was screwed on so tightly.

Then one of the leprosy patients volunteered to open the jar. Dr. Taylor handed it to him, and the patient squeezed and twisted on the lid for over a minute until his arms were shaking. He finally opened the jar and handed it back to my colleague, who noticed that the patient's hand was bleeding profusely! His leprosy blocked the pain sensations, so he kept trying because he didn't know he was hurting himself. The disease effectively blocked nerve transmission from his hands to the pain-processing circuits in his brain. The people who felt the pain stopped trying because they didn't want to hurt themselves.

Some individuals are unable to experience pain due to a condition called *congenital analgesia*. Perhaps you have seen circus performers with this genetic mutation. They are able to stick pins through their skin with no discomfort. Unfortunately, people with congenital analgesia have a severely shortened life expectancy because they lack life-saving acute pain signals to warn them of threats to their health. Pain may feel bad, but we need to appreciate its role in promoting our well-being. Pain protects us. The problem with chronic pain is that the warning signal malfunctions and goes off at the wrong times.

AN ALLEGORY FOR PAIN:
THE SIX BLIND MEN AND THE ELEPHANT

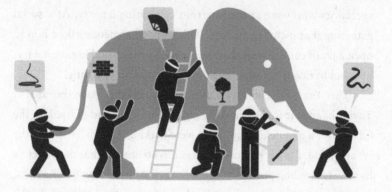

Chronic pain needs to be understood in a multifaceted way, as an interactive combination of bodily sensations, emotions, and thoughts. This integrated approach is explained well in an ancient allegory, the story of the Six Blind Men and the Elephant. The six blind men live in a remote village that has never encountered an elephant and has no concept of one. One day an elephant approaches the village, so the six blind men go out to examine the creature. Each man reaches out to feel what the animal is like, and then reports his findings to the others. One man grabs a leg and tells the others the animal resembles a large tree. Another handles the trunk and says the creature is like a large snake. One grabs the tail and says it's like a rope. Others put their hands on the tusks ("Feels like a spear"), the ears ("Feels like a giant leaf"), and the side of the animal ("Feels like a wall") and report their results. They all have contradictory descriptions of the elephant, yet they are all correct in their own ways.

It does not make sense to just consider one perspective and ignore the others. An elephant is not all about its leg or its trunk. It would be ludicrous for the six men to argue with each other, although this sort of thing happens all the time. One person is so certain of their perspective that they can't imagine that the others could also be correct. But if they cooperated, and perhaps changed places with each other, they could soon piece all the descriptions together to make a whole.

You can see that, given the complex nature of chronic pain, we need to pay attention to all of its perspectives. It is no coincidence that the three dimensions of pain roughly correlate to the three types of awareness in the ABC method: cognitive, emotional, and bodily sensation. I want you to understand pain in a comprehensive way. It is not a matter of choosing one perspective (typically, sensation) while ignoring the others. Only by integrating all the dimensions of the pain experience do we get a complete idea of it. Thus, the more completely we understand pain, the more successfully we can treat it.

Some aspects of pain are biological, some are psychological, some involve social relationships, and most involve various interactions among them. A mindset that sees the body and mind as separate things cannot understand or effectively deal with this multifaceted problem. Thanks to scientific advances in neurophysiology and other disciplines, we now realize that your mind interacts with your body through the nervous system, hormonal system, and immune system. This realization gave rise to a collaborative approach to chronic pain in the emerging field of *psychoneuroimmunology* (a combination of psychology, neurophysiology, and immunology).

To treat chronic pain effectively, we need to get an idea of how these different perspectives fit together. We will examine how your sensory experience, emotions, thoughts, and physiology are all tied together via their interplay in the body and brain.

CHAPTER 2

How Pain Works in Your Brain and Nervous System

Fans of the musical *My Fair Lady* will remember that, when Professor Henry Higgins was trying to teach articulation to Eliza, he had her repeat the phrase, "The rain in Spain lies mainly in the plain." Years ago, when I was first confronting the mysteries of pain, one of my mentors summarized the issue with a memorable paraphrase of that saying: "The gain in pain lies mainly in the brain."

My mentor's words have stuck with me because he was right. The answers to the riddle of pain are found in the brain and how it functions with regard to the body and mind. One of the immediate objectives of this book is to provide you with a greater understanding of what happens in the mind, brain, and nervous system and body in chronic pain. This knowledge will empower you and help you to better understand the confusing array of signs and symptoms that you are suffering through.

THE PAIN NETWORK IN THE BRAIN

With some eighty-six billion neurons and countless interactions between them, the human brain is far and away the most complex piece of bio-machinery on Earth. How it works is mostly a mystery, but our scientific understanding of it has increased rapidly in the last few decades because of breakthroughs in brain imaging. We can see what parts of the brain "light up" during various states of mind. The areas that are active when you feel pain are working together in what we call the pain network.

One of the most miraculous things about our brain is the way that numerous parts interact in concert with each other. In pain, for example, each area processes a different aspect of pain—such as its intensity or location—but all this information comes together to form a single experience, a unified perception. In that respect it is like a symphony orchestra. I could describe an orchestra by breaking it down to different sections: strings, horns, woodwinds, percussion—and of course the conductor. I could elaborate by describing the sounds and functions of specific instruments within those sections: oboe, viola, harp, tympani, or flute. The magic of symphonic music is the unified sound that emerges from the multitude of instruments, and the thousands of interactions between them. The whole is more than the sum of its parts.

We can understand our brain in the same way. The formation of our experience can only be understood in the context of these miraculous networks within the brain. The function of the pain network will give us a basis for understanding and treating chronic pain.

For our purposes, the brain can be divided into three main parts: brainstem, limbic system, and neocortex. The interplay of these three regions forms the neurological context of chronic pain. Their interactions also explain a lot about human behavior in general.

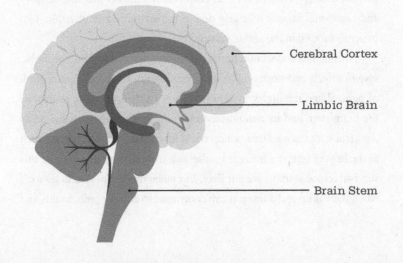

Cerebral Cortex

Limbic Brain

Brain Stem

BRAIN STEM

The brain stem regulates the most fundamental life systems of the body. It controls the heartbeat, breathing, reflexes and whether one is awake or sleepy, hungry, or sated. It is the conduit for relaying both motor and sensory nerve signals from the brain to the body, and from the body back to the brain.

LIMBIC SYSTEM

The limbic system plays a central role in forming our experience of chronic pain. The limbic system is not a separate brain structure, but rather a collection of structures that include the amygdala, hypothalamus, hippocampus, and insula. In concert they inspect and evaluate incoming sensory signals, including pain signals. The sensory information is compared to past memories and assigned an emotional value. The entire bundle of sensory and emotional information is then forwarded to other parts of the brain.

The intensity of the emotions attached to pain signals determines how disruptive the pain can be. As I mentioned earlier, the International Association for the Study of Pain (IASP) defines pain as, "An unpleasant sensory and emotional experience associated with···actual or potential tissue damage." The reason that pain is defined as combining sensory and emotional factors is largely due to the anatomy and physiology of structures found in the limbic system.

Through its connection to the autonomic nervous system, the limbic system affects our hormonal system, our digestion, and our perception of pain. When the limbic system perceives a threat, it seizes control of the brain stem and its autonomic functions. In a situation evaluated as dangerous, an intense fear reaction could set off a defense mechanism such as the fight–flight–or–freeze response. In a truly dangerous situation, this survival response may save our lives. But when this alarm system goes off when there is no real danger, it can contribute to chronic pain. In this and other ways, the limbic system affects how we experience pain in terms of its intensity, intrusiveness, and level of distress.

The limbic system merits special attention when it comes to understanding the experience of chronic pain. Its profound influence on the autonomic nervous system and its effects on sensory information, emotional information, and memory make it a power to be reckoned with. We will address how to address an overactive limbic system later in the book, in a section called "Limbic Retraining" (see Chapter 22 in section V).

NEOCORTEX (CEREBRAL CORTEX)

The neocortex is the big wrinkly covering you see when you look at a picture of a brain. The term *cortex* is from a Latin word meaning bark, the outermost layer. In addition to being the most prominent visible feature of the brain, it is also the most highly evolved part. It is the seat of cognition, consciousness, and language—the place where we think, imagine, and plan.

The four lobes of the cerebral cortex are responsible for three main functions:

1. Sensation

2. Motor activity

3. Association

The *sensory* areas of the cerebral cortex receive information from the body about touch-related sensations like pain and temperature. The *motor* areas are involved in initiating movement in the body. This is the source of our voluntary control over moving our arms and legs and other body parts. The *association* areas integrate information from multiple brain regions to form unified perceptions, rather than a random pile of sensory data. For example, the visual association cortex will take the basic aspects of a visual image—such as color, shape, and size—and put them all together to create a perception of an object that is composed of those diverse elements. Instead of seeing patches of blue and different angles from the right eye and left eye, all that information is integrated so that you see, for example, a book on a table six feet away.

At the front of the cerebral cortex, right behind your forehead, is an area called the *prefrontal cortex* or PFC. The PFC can help to inhibit, delay, or correct dysfunctional or impulsive reactions. It is the part of the brain that can remind you to count to ten, so you don't lose your temper and react to something out of anger. It reminds you to take a deep breath when a strong feeling of fear overtakes you. It is the place that reminds you, when you are startled by the sound of a civil defense siren, that it's just the monthly test of the system and not a warning of severe weather or some other emergency. In this way the "wise moderator" can assign a less threatening meaning to an event and downregulate emotional reactions.

KEY AREAS IN THE PAIN NETWORK

The components of the pain network function within and across the three main parts of the brain. Let's turn up the detail on our microscope and take a look at some of the individual areas along the pain network to see how they contribute to our feeling of pain.

THALAMUS: *THE SENSORY RELAY CENTER*

The thalamus is the relay station of the brain. Almost all sensory information flows from the spinal cord up through the thalamus. The thalamus distributes these signals to all other parts of the brain. For example, signals go to the amygdala in the limbic system to assign emotional significance to them and to judge whether they pose a threat. The signals are also sent to sensory areas of the cerebral cortex to identify the signal in terms of sensation, pain, or temperature.

AMYGDALA: *THE SECURITY GUARD*

The amygdala is the part of the brain responsible for watching out for threats. It automatically evaluates the sense data it receives from the thalamus, and attaches an emotional significance to them. It also affects memories of emotionally charged events. When the amygdala scans sensory signals that indicate danger, it can activate the autonomic nervous system.

Imagine the amygdala as a security guard whose job it is to keep an eye on a group of monitors from security cameras throughout a big building. He is constantly checking to see if anything is wrong. If a problem shows up on a monitor, such as a burglar breaking in, he will set off the alarms. The alarm triggers the fight–flight–or–freeze reaction through the autonomic nervous system.

But what if somebody plays a trick on our security guard and brings in an actor made up to look like a burglar? This security guard is easily fooled and will sound the alarm just the same.

Likewise, our amygdala sometimes signals alarm in situations that are not necessarily dangerous. People who struggle with post–traumatic stress disorder (PTSD) suffer with this. For example, consider a soldier who has fought in combat, experiencing the horrors of war and witnessing violent injury and death. Years later, he is back home, walking down the street. He hears a car's engine backfire, and he immediately dives for cover. His amygdala is signaling a threat where there isn't one.

The amygdala doesn't know the difference between an *actual* event and the *image* or *memory* of an event, and will create the same physiological response. It is very important to understand how this internal error affects your experience of chronic pain.

HIPPOCAMPUS: *REMEMBER THIS*

The hippocampus encodes incoming sensory information for storage in longer–term memory. It also integrates this information, combining sensations, sights, sounds, smells, and tastes. When you think about your son or daughter, the memory you retrieve of them is mixed in with various sensory data—how they look, perhaps the smell of the shampoo or cologne they use, as well as various emotions that you feel toward them. It all comes together in one package.

The hippocampus also determines which pieces of sensory information are important and worth remembering. Memories with strong emotional reactions tend to stand out. For example, you probably don't remember what you had for lunch two weeks ago, but you likely remember where you were on September 11, 2001. This phenomenon is also true for the memory of painful sensations.

The problem for chronic pain sufferers is that the proper function of the hippocampus can be hampered by stress. That's because it has a high concentration of receptor sites for stress hormones, such as cortisol, and other similar neurohormones. When it is under stress, the hippocampus can distort both the encoding and recall of memories. Memories of pain in a particular part of the body can be experienced and recalled differently, depending on how much the amygdala and hippocampus identify it as stressful.

INSULA: *WHERE IS MY BODY IN SPACE?*

The insula integrates the sensory and emotional aspects of pain perception with its sense of the body in space and control of motor movements. The combined result is our feeling of suffering as part of the pain experience. I have seen how this plays out many times, where a pain sensation will change a person's behavior. Let's say someone who is suffering from abdominal pain has plans to see a friend. But then they get a slight twinge of pain in their gut, so they cancel the date.

ANTERIOR CINGULATE CORTEX: *JUST HOW BAD IS THIS PAIN?*

The anterior cingulate cortex (ACC) evaluates pain sensations with a focus on the pain's emotional aspects. Emotional responses cause the ACC to become more highly activated, which makes the pain feel worse. Research has shown that the ACC becomes more highly activated in patients with chronic pain, increasing the effect of the production of pain.

Emotion plays such a strong role in the ACC because it is highly interconnected with the amygdala and hypothalamus. This makes it a player in the regulation of emotional experience and assigning emotions to various sensations. It also increases verbal expression about the difficulty and struggle associated with a painful episode. This is why someone with chronic pain can be overwhelmed with feelings of panic, frustration, or despair after feeling a twinge of pain.

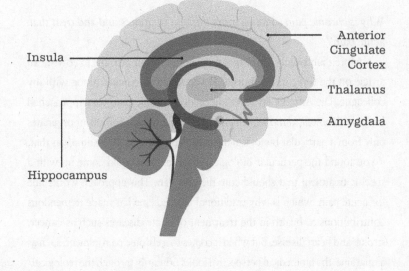

Insula

Hippocampus

Anterior
Cingulate
Cortex

Thalamus

Amygdala

CHAPTER 3

Two Kinds of Pain—
Acute and Chronic

Why is chronic pain so much more difficult to understand and treat than acute pain?

More than twenty years ago, this question prompted me to cowrite an article on the topic in the journal *Postgraduate Medicine*, along with my colleague, Dr. Alfred Clavel. Traditionally, chronic pain was approached from the *biomedical model*, which holds that any pain complaint originates only from a particular biological disorder. The thinking at the time was that, if you found the particular biological disorder, you could come up with a specific treatment that should cure the problem. This approach works fine for acute pain, which is why traditional biomedicine has made tremendous contributions to health in the treatment of acute diseases such as cancer, stroke, and heart disease. But when it comes to a chronic pain ailment, such as a migraine, the biomedical perspective looks primarily through the biological/biomechanical "windows" and thus has difficulties understanding the rest. What we have is a paradigm that is valid as far as it goes—but it's incomplete.

In order to properly treat chronic pain, we need to understand how it works and how it differs from acute pain. Their names tell a lot. Chronic means long-lasting, and acute means more recent. Chronic lasts for a long time, from three to six months to begin with, and it can continue for years. Acute pain arises sharply from an injury or a disease of recent origin, but it is over relatively quickly, too. Acute pain is generally associated with tissue damage—a biological problem—and the pain tells you where it is in your body. "I hurt my foot!" or, "There's a sharp pain on my left side." The physician examines the extent of any damage and prescribes the appropriate treatment, which often includes pain medications—which are quite effective against acute pain. When the damage has healed, the acute pain goes away.

By contrast, chronic pain may persist long after the initial injuries have healed. Chronic pain symptoms are not always a reliable indicator for tracking down the cause of the pain. Remember Janice? Her back still hurt even after her ruptured disc had healed.

Examples of Ailments Associated with Each Type of Pain	
ACUTE PAIN	**CHRONIC PAIN**
Bee sting	Chronic back or neck pain
Broken bone	Chronic migraine/ tension headache
Burns	Osteoarthritis
Appendicitis	Fibromyalgia
Stubbed toe	Irritable bowel syndrome (IBS)
Childbirth	Chronic muscle tension
A cut	Chronic temporomandibular disorders (TMD)
Getting punched in the stomach	Chronic rheumatoid arthritis
Toothache	Chronic acid reflux (gastroesophageal reflux disease—GERD)

SIMPLE VERSUS COMPLEX PAIN

Another important distinction between the two types of pain is that acute pain is more simple and chronic pain is more complex. Likewise, the treatments for acute pain are more straightforward, while treating chronic pain is much more complicated. Look at the difference between a broken leg and a migraine headache. There's no mystery why your leg hurts: You broke a bone. The treatment is well-established. Put your leg in a cast and take some ibuprofen.

Compare that to a migraine headache, which can have a dozen contributing factors, ranging from an oversensitized central nervous system to various types of stress. For migraines and other types of chronic pain, painkillers become less effective over time. Some pain medicines, like opioids, start making the pain worse when taken over time.

The impact of emotion differs in acute pain versus chronic pain. In acute pain, emotions are less likely to contribute to maintaining or worsening the symptoms. Emotion can affect the intensity of the pain, and the intensity of your reaction to the injury. For example, if you sprain your ankle the day before your dance recital, there will be a good deal of anguish. But if you sprain your ankle and it gets you out of a boring business trip to Boise, you almost feel lucky to have been injured. Emotions aside, you would still follow the same health care routine: Go to the clinic and have it examined. They'd take X-rays to make sure you didn't fracture a bone. You'd receive treatment until the tendon or the fracture healed, and then you'd be done. The pain would recede, and with it, the anger or anxiety.

In chronic pain, however, emotion plays a central and much more important role. Emotional suffering can become a key part of the cycle of chronic pain. The very presence of chronic pain disrupts one's lifestyle, and that causes emotional turmoil. In turn, those negative emotions physically worsen the condition and help to perpetuate chronic pain. This is no coincidence, because many of the areas in the brain that process emotion also process pain.

The complexity of migraines and other sorts of chronic pain creates a formidable puzzle for both patient and provider. When a physician cannot tie your report of pain to tissue damage, they may be stumped as to what direction to take. After well-meaning clinicians conduct all the likely tests and try various treatments that don't help, they may conclude the problem is psychosomatic.

Patients are stumped as well, so they keep looking for second opinions, and go to various specialists seeking help. When all the tests and treatments don't work, the repeated failures take an emotional toll on the patient. As time goes on, their despair and frustration grow to be as debilitating as the pain itself. They cut back on their activities, socialize less, and have lower productivity. A restricted lifestyle dominated by chronic pain leaves a person feeling trapped, miserable, and hopeless.

Many pain treatments don't work because they were designed for acute pain, not chronic pain. In order to formulate appropriate treatment plans, we must address the underlying challenges that are *unique to chronic pain*. Typically, there are no quick answers because chronic pain is complicated, and these complications need to be understood. As an example of this complexity, let's take a look at twelve factors that contribute to migraine, which is representative of many kinds of chronic pain.

POSSIBLE CONTRIBUTING FACTORS
FOR MIGRAINE HEADACHES

1. **Genetic vulnerability to the condition:** For some people, the disposition to get migraines is built-in at birth.

2. **Neurogenic inflammation:** Certain nerves release substances that initiate an inflammatory reaction. This can result in swelling, tenderness, and pain.

3. **Co-occurring physical conditions** such as *temporomandibular* disorders (TMD), which cause facial pain or tenderness in the jawbone and the temple/skull area.

4. **Central sensitization syndrome (CSS)**: a condition in which the central nervous system—the brain and spinal cord—become overly sensitized to pain signals. We will discuss CSS more fully on page 49.

5. **Autonomic dysregulation**: An imbalance in the autonomic nervous system between the sympathetic and parasympathetic subsystems. We will discuss autonomic dysregulation more fully in the next few chapters.

6. **Dietary stress**: Negative bodily reactions to what we eat or drink, such as food allergies or gluten intolerance.

7. **Myofascial tightness, instability, and trigger points**: Painful knots caused by irritations in the muscles and connective tissue.

8. **External stress triggers**: Problems dealing with work, home, relationships, financial stress, etc.

9. **Internal stress triggers**: Problems in your inner life, including ongoing chronic emotional conflicts, ongoing depression or anxiety, or post-traumatic stress reactions.

10. **Environmental stressors**: Atmospheric conditions such as barometric pressure, temperature changes, or chemical sensitivities.

11. **Analgesic rebound**: A dynamic reversal of the effects of pain medications—they start to *increase* pain rather than decrease it—following extended use of the analgesic.

12. **Adverse or allergic reactions to certain medications**: Everything from hives and itching to anaphylactic (allergic) shock.

Here is where we must hark back to the allegory of the Six Blind Men and the Elephant. The first challenge is to understand the complexity as a whole. The six blind men found six diverse body parts that were unified in a single elephant. An elephant cannot be reduced to its leg or its trunk. We can stand back and see how the parts of an elephant are conjoined into a single animal. Similarly, we can begin to see how chronic pain can have diverse aspects, such as environmental stressors, medication rebound, depression, allergies, genetic predispositions, and nervous system dysregulation.

Differences in Acute Pain vs. Chronic Pain

DEFINITIONS

- Acute pain is the ordinary pain that accompanies tissue damage; it is a usually a sharp pain that comes on quickly and is gone within a few weeks to a month or two

- Chronic pain lasts at least three to six months

THE FEELING OF PAIN

- Subjectively, acute pain and chronic pain may feel the same

THE FUNCTION OF PAIN

- Acute pain is usually a reliable symptom indicator of actual or possible tissue damage

- Chronic pain is usually not a reliable symptom indicator of tissue damage

DURATION

- Acute pain is temporary; it goes away after the tissue damage has healed

- Chronic pain can linger for years, even after the site of initial injury has healed

ROLE OF EMOTIONS

- Emotions may occur in response to acute pain, but rarely affect the course of the pain

- Emotions and other psychological states can be dominant factors in complicating chronic pain

COMPLEXITY

- Acute pain is relatively simple
- Chronic pain is usually more complex

PAIN MEDICATIONS

- Acute pain generally responds well to pain medications
- Chronic pain may not respond well to pain medications: some painkillers actually increase feelings of pain

TREATMENT APPROACH

- Acute pain can be effectively treated by a primary care provider
- Most often, chronic pain is best treated by a team approach that includes a physician, clinical psychologist, physical therapist, and other clinicians

CHAPTER 4

How Chronic Pain Changes the Nervous System— Central Sensitization and Autonomic Dysregulation

CENTRAL SENSITIZATION SYNDROME (CSS)

In chronic pain, when pain lasts longer than three to six months, the nervous system changes both physically and functionally. One of the important contributions to our understanding of chronic pain is the idea of the central sensitization syndrome (CSS), formulated by Muhammad B. Yunus. He discovered that, regardless of the original cause of the pain, if pain signals travel repeatedly down a neuron over an extended time period, it tends to become oversensitized. When nociceptors—the neurons that carry pain signals—get sensitized, a neurochemical reaction takes place. The nervous system goes through a process called *wind-up*, escalating into a persistent state of high reactivity. This persistent reactivity makes everything feel more painful and may transmit the feeling of pain even after the initial injury has healed.

There are two basic forms of heightened sensitivity in CSS:

1. **Hyperalgesia**—Literally, "increased pain." When this occurs, a stimulus that may be painful is perceived as much more painful than it should be. For example, turning your head when you have a stiff neck may ordinarily be mildly painful, but with hyperalgesia, this pain will feel excruciating.

2. **Allodynia**—Literally, "other pain." This is a condition in which non-painful stimuli cause pain. For example, a slight touch on the hand may feel extraordinarily painful. Since the nerve is damaged, it may recruit nearby nerves to help with its work of carrying pain signals. Consequently, a nerve that ordinarily carries touch sensations may send pain signals when someone is touched. Since the nervous system is in a persistent state of high reactivity, the brain produces a sensation of pain rather than a mild sensation of touch.

CSS can also lead to increased sensitivities across all of the senses, not just the sense of touch. The chronic pain sufferer may report sensitivity to odors, sounds, or light. Sometimes a bright light or a whiff of perfume can be enough to set off a headache. CSS is also associated with increased emotional distress. Remember, the nervous system handles both sensations and emotions. CSS has become widely recognized as important in many chronic pain disorders.

It is estimated that at least 70 percent of patients with chronic back pain referred to pain clinics exhibit features of CSS, which go beyond the local, structural causes of pain such as a slipped disc, pulled muscles, etc.

Over my thirty-three years of working in a chronic pain clinic, I observed that many patients who came in with a chronic headache or low back pain also had a cluster of common problems:

- TMD—jaw pain known as temporomandibular disorder

- IBS—irritable bowel syndrome

- Chronic neck pain

- Chronic fatigue syndrome

- Fibromyalgia—chronic widespread pain

- Multiple chemical sensitivity

Later, as I read the research of Yunus and others, I realized that CSS might be the common denominator among these complaints. For example, about 40 percent of the patients who came in for facial pain, headache, or low back pain also complained of IBS and other digestive distress. This led to my interest in treating abdominal pain such as IBS, eventually culminating in my book *Trust Your Gut* (Conari Press, 2013).

AUTONOMIC DYSREGULATION

Beyond the central nervous system—the brain and spinal cord—lies the peripheral nervous system (PNS). These nerves branch out to the organs and every part of the body. An important component of the PNS is the autonomic nervous system (ANS), which automatically regulates involuntary physical processes—like heart rate, blood pressure, respiration, digestion, and sexual arousal. The autonomic system works outside of your conscious awareness to control basic functions. You don't have to think about it for these processes to work.

The ANS plays an important role in responding to stress. Working in tandem with other physiological processes, the ANS helps us respond to any stressors that may interfere with our well-being and ultimate survival.

When it is functioning properly, the ANS helps to maintain that balance during stressful events. But when the ANS itself gets out of balance, it can't do its job. When this happens, it ends up adding stress instead of relieving it. This harmful state is called *autonomic dysregulation*, and it occurs commonly among people with chronic pain.

The two main components of the ANS are the sympathetic and the parasympathetic branches. The sympathetic branch is activating—think of it as the gas pedal. It is associated with energy mobilization in situations requiring intense physical and/or mental effort. In its extreme, it helps carry out the fight-or-flight response, where quick reactions are needed. The parasympathetic branch plays the opposite role—think of it as the brake pedal. The parasympathetic branch is all about "rest and digest." It slows down our system, allowing for relaxation and recovery after exertion.

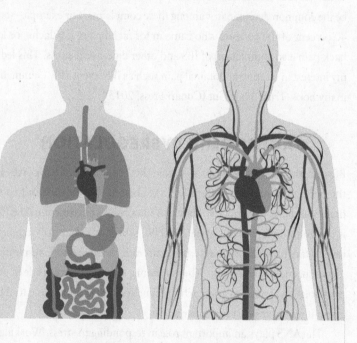

SYMPATHETIC
activation

heart rate ↑
salivary flow ↓
stomach motility ↓
stress horomones ↑

PARASYMPATHETIC
activation

↓ heart rate
↑ salivary flow
↑ stomach motility
↓ stress horomones

The sympathetic and parasympathetic systems are engaged in a constant dance, an ongoing balancing act. We all experience normal cycles of activity and rest, periods of excitement followed by times of calm, high-energy activities giving way to times of low energy and rest. Even as we slumber, the sympathetic and parasympathetic systems do their balancing duet as we alternate through deeper and lighter levels of sleep. For many cultures, the natural cycle of low activity is marked by the *siesta*—the afternoon nap. When sympathetic and parasympathetic periods are in relative balance, we feel good and all is well. The pendulum is well-oiled, swinging back and forth.

But when the ANS is out of balance and the equilibrium is disturbed, the playful dance becomes a tug-of-war. All is not well when the pendulum gets stuck. The dominance of either branch causes dysregulation, but it is most often commonly a hyperactive sympathetic system. The foot gets stuck on the gas. Or the pendulum can swing more wildly to extremes: Very intense agitation alternates with profound exhaustion and depletion. In fact, I sometimes describe this predicament to my patients as being like "having your foot on the gas pedal and the brake at the same time." Areas of physical vulnerability are weakened further and distress is heightened. Autonomic dysregulation intensifies and perpetuates chronic pain.

WHAT EXACTLY HAPPENS WHEN THE ANS GETS DYSREGULATED?

Think of how your body responds to perceived danger. It could be anything from the sound of footsteps behind you in a dark alley to an oncoming car with blinding headlights, or a twinge of burning pain streaking down your leg. When these things spark fear, your survival mode switches on.

Traditionally, we think of three classic responses: fight, flight, or freeze. These responses automatically cause hormonal and physiological changes that allow you to act quickly for self-protection. These reactions are not consciously chosen. Everything happens too fast, before you have time to think.

The amygdala sounds the alarm when it senses a serious threat, fulfilling its role as the primary fear–perception center in your brain. The amygdala sends signals to your hypothalamus, the ringleader of the stress–response system called the HPA axis. The hypothalamus sets off the ANS, prompting the release of stress hormones such as adrenaline and cortisol. Fight and flight reactions increase heart rate, speed up breathing, and make your vision and hearing hyperalert and vigilant to potential threats. The freeze response produces decreased heart rate, and breathing becomes slower and more restricted.

An event that illustrates the gamut of fight, flight, and freeze reactions is the trauma of September 11, 2001. As we watched the horrifying images of the Twin Towers in lower Manhattan that morning on TV, different types of responses were apparent. The fight response was represented by the throngs of people who were protesting like an angry mob. They shook their fists in the air and vowed to attack whoever did this. The flight response was obvious in the masses of people running across the Brooklyn Bridge, fleeing from the World Trade Center. Finally, there were large groups of people who illustrated the freeze response. They stood motionless just a couple blocks away from the smoke and flames. They were stunned and simply stared in numb disbelief. Fight, flight, and freeze.

HOW DO YOU KNOW IF YOU ARE EXPERIENCING CENTRAL SENSITIZATION AND/OR AUTONOMIC DYSREGULATION?

First of all, CSS and autonomic dysregulation are more likely if you have been experiencing pain for three to six months or longer. One sign is experiencing problems with insomnia—either trouble falling asleep or trouble staying asleep at night. Ongoing anxiety or depression could be indicators. Cognitive problems could appear—often described as brain fog—when one has difficulty with concentration, attention, and memory. You may be particularly sensitive to certain sensations, such as loud noises, bright lights, smells (especially chemical smells such as paint or perfume), polluted air, temperature fluctuations, or touch (allodynia, where normal touch feels painful). Finally, you may be extremely sensitive to medications.

CHAPTER 5

Additional Concepts to Help You Understand Your Chronic Pain

Now that you have learned about how your nervous system changes because of ongoing suffering, I want to introduce some additional concepts of importance for understanding how your chronic pain works.

GATE CONTROL THEORY: *HOW TO OPEN OR CLOSE THE PAIN GATE*

Gate control theory was established from important research by psychologist Ronald Melzack and neuroscientist Patrick Wall. Before their work, it was assumed that nerve signals rise up automatically from the point of injury—such as fingers on a hot stove. It was thought they simply flow up the spinal cord to the brain, causing the experience of pain. Melzack and Wall found that there are other factors on that pathway that will either increase or decrease the pain signal. They called it the pain gate, because it can be opened or closed.

We are all familiar with this phenomenon. This is why it hurts when you accidentally hit your thumb with a hammer, but it feels better when you rub your thumb. The signals that carry the sensation of touch from the rubbing inhibit the pain signal, which dials down the pain gate, reducing the experience of pain. Likewise, the pain from an "owie" on a child's finger can go away altogether when the mother kisses it. The sensation of that gentle kiss, combined with the soothing feeling of Mom's love, closed the pain gate!

The list of factors that can open or close the pain gate is long, but each one of them suggests new opportunities for treating pain more broadly. Here is a partial list of the variables that can influence the pain gate:

- Emotions
- Expectations of pain
- Thoughts
- Attitudes toward pain
- Beliefs
- Age
- Memories of previous pain
- Sex
- Family teaching
- Social/cultural experiences
- Experiences of pain
- Sleep

Gate control theory teaches us that the experience of chronic pain is not simply a physical or biomechanical phenomenon. We now know that emotions, beliefs, family history, and cultural traditions can affect your degree of distress, which means they are also important for healing.

HPA AXIS: *YOUR BODY'S STRESS READINESS SYSTEM*

HPA stands for hypothalamus, pituitary gland, and adrenal gland. This stress–response system links the body's nervous system and the endocrine/hormonal system. It allows electrical signals to trigger the release of hormones.

- **Hypothalamus**—a part of the brain located in the limbic system

- **Pituitary gland**—a part of the endocrine system located at the base of the limbic system, below the hypothalamus

- **Adrenal gland**—a part of the endocrine system located on top of the kidneys

The HPA axis is one of our primary survival systems in the body. Its job is to prepare the body for action whenever we confront an actual (or potential) threat. Let's say you encounter something stressful. It could be an *external stress*, something you confront in your environment. In our primitive days, it could have been a bear coming toward you, or an enemy from another tribe. In our civilized world, it could be a host of fearful things:

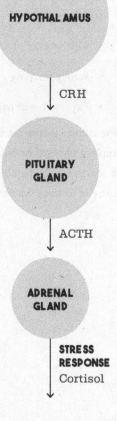

- Seeing a strange shadow outside your window at night

- Getting stopped by a policeman

- Seeing a threatening letter that your expensive utility bill is overdue

- Your boss catching you playing video games at work

Or it could be an *internal stress,* such as:

- An anxious anticipation of your spouse being annoyed with you

- Your insecure fear that your friends will reject you

- The perception of that nagging chronic pain in your neck and shoulders

Whether the source of stress is external or internal, it makes no difference to your brain. It does not matter whether the threat could actually harm your body, or merely wound your sense of pride—either way, the HPA axis responds with the release of stress hormones that activate your body. Your heart rate picks up, energy goes to your muscles, and your mind perks up with greater alertness. You are ready to respond, be it fight, flight, or freeze.

Chronic pain is one of those ongoing stressful conditions that can cause the HPA axis to malfunction. The tremendous exhaustion and burnout felt by chronic pain sufferers may be caused by an overworked HPA axis, as well as by the constant pain.

Many of the self-care strategies I will show you can calm the HPA axis so it responds more appropriately to stress, thereby reducing your pain, stress, and exhaustion.

NEUROPLASTICITY: *NEURONS THAT FIRE TOGETHER WIRE TOGETHER*

Let's break down this term: *Neuro* refers to nerves. *Plasticity* means the capacity to be molded or changed. Neuroplasticity is the inherent ability of your brain and nervous system to adapt and change. Scientists used to believe that the neural connections in our brain were hardwired and fixed by the time we reached young adulthood. It was assumed that if you suffered nerve damage, you could never replace the broken connection.

By the 1970s, researchers concluded that this belief was false. We now know that the capacity for the brain to change persists from childhood all the way to old age. The changeable nature of the nervous system has important implications for medical science. In the treatment of nerve damage, for example, it has set higher goals for recovery. Previously, practitioners looked at brain damage as a dead end, believing that no recovery was possible. But then it was discovered that electric stimulation and other treatments could train undamaged nerves to take over the work of the damaged circuit. Through repeated effort, new neural circuits could be formed. This is why physical therapy, speech therapy, and occupational therapy are standard treatments after someone suffers a stroke. Neuroplasticity enables the brain and nervous system to readily adapt to changes in the body and the external environment. Another area related to neuroplasticity is the formation of habits, for good or for ill.

One of the earliest explanations of how neuroplasticity works was offered by Canadian neuropsychologist Donald Hebb. He proposed that a communication channel between two nerve cells is strengthened when the two neurons fire simultaneously. Practicing a new behavior causes two nerves to fire together, and the connection between these nerves is strengthened. His discovery is summed up by the phrase "Neurons that fire together wire together."

This means that, when we learn a new skill or think repetitive thoughts, the neurons that keep firing together are more likely to form lasting patterns. This is true with conscious learning—such as learning a new language—as well as subconscious learning, such as reacting instinctively to the sound of someone's voice.

For better or for worse, we humans are habit-forming creatures. There are both positive and negative consequences of this ability to create neural habits. You experience positive neuroplasticity every day when you learn to do something beneficial automatically, without conscious effort. When you first learn to drive a car, you have to pay attention to every little detail when you make a turn or stop. But after driving a lot, these skills become second nature. Eventually, you can drive home on automatic pilot, without needing to use Google Maps. Positive neuroplasticity makes things easier.

Neuroplasticity is important for the chronic pain sufferer because negative neuroplasticity makes things more difficult. One example is how repeated pain signals can damage nerves, causing them to become hypersensitive. This is the basis of central sensitization (CSS). Once this occurs, normal movement and tasks become painful when they shouldn't be.

Another example of negative neuroplasticity is the bad habit formed when someone with chronic low back pain starts to walk with a limp. The person tries to guard against further pain by bracing their muscles. But then their pelvis, legs, and feet start to move in an unbalanced fashion. Over time, the resultant limp becomes a habit, as parts of the nervous system start to wire together. The result is even greater pain and distress. For those of you who have suffered hip, back, or leg pain and sought physical therapy, you'll now understand why the physical therapist emphasized the importance of you walking without a limp.

Negative neuroplasticity may bring with it a host of unwanted effects:

- Withdrawing from useful activities like work or physical exercise

- Poor sleep

- Low mood

- Increased stress and pain behaviors

- Being less able or willing to engage in activities to take care of yourself

The good news is that *positive* neuroplasticity can be taught. It is possible to reeducate your brain and nervous system through the repeated practice of some specific exercises. This is why regular practice of self-care exercises is so very important and helpful: Repetitive practice encourages the formation of positive new neural pathways. This will enable you to resume your everyday activities without fearing to do so. We will introduce these healing exercises in the next chapter of this book, my treatment recommendations.

INFLAMMATION:
BOTH A HERO AND A VILLAIN

Inflammation can be both a savior and a curse when it comes to your health. On the positive side, inflammation is a natural defense against disease, provided by the immune system. When you are injured or get an infection, your body releases hormones that tell the immune system to send white blood cells to the affected areas to repair the injury or fight infection. You may have noticed that when a cut gets infected, the surrounding area gets warm, red, and swollen. This is the process of inflammation at work to heal you. When an injury or infection heals, inflammation normally disappears.

However, sometimes this healing process gets stuck in the activation mode and does not go away. Instead of helping you, it becomes chronic inflammation that can damage healthy cells and organs. It can also contribute to chronic pain in muscles, tissues, and joints. Stress, particularly when chronic, is associated with an overactive immune system. Additionally, the nervous system can also manifest a type of inflammation called *neurogenic inflammation*. Neurogenic inflammation increases sensitization throughout the body, which makes you more vulnerable to experiencing chronic pain.

This relationship between the immune system and inflammation is important to understanding what happens in chronic pain. When pain is chronic (lasting more than three to six months), pro-inflammatory immune cells secrete chemicals called *cytokines*, which signal the nervous system to become more inflamed. This is a central element of how inflammation in the nervous system increases both central sensitization (CSS) and autonomic (ANS) dysregulation. Recent research suggests that *glial cells* are important in understanding why the immune system mistakenly sends signals that cause increased inflammation in the nervous system.

The sympathetic/parasympathetic balance of the ANS affects the extent to which the flames of chronic inflammation are either fanned or cooled down. That means that the levels of stress we experience have a direct effect on inflammation and chronic pain.

Happily, there are all kinds of things you can do to reduce inflammation and the pain that can result from it. Several of the skills I will provide you, including calming techniques, exercise, pacing, stress management, and dietary changes, can help reduce chronic inflammation. We will discuss these techniques in the next chapter.

STATE-DEPENDENT MEMORY & CHRONIC PAIN: *MEMORIES IN FULL TECHNICOLOR*

If you suffer from chronic pain, you have most likely experienced negative state-dependent memory. The concept of state-dependent memory emerged over the past century in memory research. Early studies found that people can recall more information when they are in the same physical or mental state as they were in the original experience. A common example is someone who lost their keys while intoxicated. They couldn't remember where they put their keys when they got sober, but when they got drunk again it all came back to them!

Another aspect of state-dependent memory has much greater relevance for chronic pain. This is where something in the present moment triggers a vivid memory, and it all comes rushing back to you like a flashback in a movie.

Some years ago, I flew to Switzerland for the first time. As we were about to land in Geneva, I was listening to some music by a great a cappella jazz group called Take 6. Now, every time I hear their haunting harmonies, it brings me back to all the wonderful experiences from that Swiss trip. I get a heart-pounding flash of excitement and anticipation, vivid images of lush green trees and blue water, and a sense of eager anticipation. I don't just remember it—*I'm there.*

We've all experienced how the fragrance of a certain flower or the sound of a favorite song can send us back to some past moment. Try a little experiment. Close your eyes for a moment. Now picture the face of someone you love. Feel the warmth in your heart. Sense that smile that just won't quit. This is *positive* state-dependent memory. It brings back good feelings.

A good example of positive state-dependent memory is when you get a whiff of freshly baked cookies and suddenly you are back in your grandma's kitchen. You can see her pulling the cookies out of the oven and pouring you a glass of cold milk. Is your mouth watering? You're not just remembering it—you're there! State-dependent memory is a hologram of sensations, images, emotions, behavioral impulses—all experienced in full Technicolor.

But it works both ways. A random sensory cue can also trigger painful experiences from the past. This we call *negative* state-dependent memory.

Several months ago, a friend of mine was using a drill to repair a shovel and he accidentally drilled into his middle finger. Ouch! The bit went right through his finger! The pain was excruciating, not to mention all the blood. Now, whenever he thinks about that horrible moment, his finger starts throbbing. He'll walk into his workshop and see the drill—and "Ouch!" He hears the moment the drill bit went through his finger—he sees the blood—and he absolutely feels the pain. He doesn't just "remember it"—he *relives* the whole multisensory experience!

Negative state-dependent memory is very common in chronic pain, but is rarely recognized in its diagnosis or treatment. I have found that state-dependent memories are often an important factor when we examine the complex web of chronic pain.

For many people, the experience of chronic back pain, neck pain, headache, etc., may trigger a cascade of negative emotions such as anger, sadness, despair, or rage. Negative images can surface. You picture yourself in the future as a hopeless wreck. You limp along, unable to do the things you always loved—like biking or going on a long hike. This just adds more pain and tension to what you already feel. Negative thoughts may resurface from the original painful event. You think to yourself, "I'm so mad at myself for not feeling well. What's wrong with my body? It's hopeless to even think about getting better!"

As you are reliving this terrible experience from the past, your amygdala reacts as if it is a current event, and it sets off the alarm. Memories of the original event get associated with the severe pain you felt at the time. For example, if your pain originated in a car accident where your head jerked forward at the moment of impact, whenever you move your head forward—even years into the future—it brings back quite vividly the pain and fear of the moment when you were hurt.

A FATHERLY FLASHBACK

Bill was a chronic pain patient in his late forties who had a disruptive state-dependent memory that dated back to his childhood. Bill suffered from a neuropathic condition that caused a burning electrical pain in his left leg. But, quite curiously, every time the pain struck, Bill immediately launched into a highly emotional state of anger, agitation, and shame. When I zeroed in on this unusual response to his pain, Bill ultimately revealed that the pain was sparking an old memory. When Bill was a child, his father was an alcoholic who never kept a job longer than a month or two. Instead of taking responsibility for his joblessness, his father always blamed his alleged "bad health." He would always repeat that lousy excuse for not working harder. Bill said, "When I feel my leg pain, it makes me feel ashamed. I'm afraid that I am just like my father."

Once we identified this negative state-dependent reaction, Bill could begin to interrupt this cycle that unwittingly maintained his suffering.

Keep in mind that state-dependent memory is just that—a memory. It is not the reality of the present moment. When chronic pain pulls you into a negative state-dependent memory, it dissociates you from the present. It is an inherent state of disconnection. Recognizing the cruel trick of negative state-dependent memory is an important step in healing from chronic pain.

Later in the book, we will discuss several helpful tools for healing negative state-dependent memories.

CHAPTER 6

Why Medications Don't Work as Well for Chronic Pain

It seems that many people have at least one medication that they rely on. "Two of these little pills really took care of my back pain," or "My sister got fast relief from this, so now I want to take this drug too," or "I finally found my wonder drug. What allergies? They disappeared!" This kind of adulation for medications makes you want to think that there's always a drug solution for any problem. The reality is, the story on chronic pain is far more complex. It is a widespread but mistaken notion that medications can be the primary treatment for chronic pain.

MEDICATIONS CAN PLAY A HELPFUL ROLE

I am not saying that pain medications can't play a role in the treatment of chronic pain. From an integrative medicine orientation, medications can be one part of a broader healing plan. For example, the time-limited use of analgesic pain medication and muscle relaxants may break the pain cycle just long enough for the patient to begin to feel a little relief and take the first steps toward self-care activities. Sometimes the short-term use of a benzodiazepine (tranquilizer) may allow the patient to know what it feels like for a chronically tight muscle to begin to relax. This "experiential reference point" may then help the patient to navigate on his own during the journey to calm his muscles and nervous system. Sometimes the judicious use of an anticonvulsant medication such as gabapentin (Neurontin) or pregabalin (Lyrica) may be helpful in the early stages of treatment, for helping to make the pain symptoms less overwhelming and intrusive. And sometimes antidepressant medication may help a chronic pain sufferer break the pain–depression–anxiety–tensing cycle long enough to "untie their hands" from behind their back and use their other coping strategies more successfully.

A patient of mine who suffered from chronic low back pain and depression described his experience of how medications fit in to the overall treatment with this apt metaphor:

"My chronic low back pain and depression felt to me like trying to start a fire when the wood was wet. For me, the pain medication and antidepressant medication were like dry kindling, helping me to get the fire started. But the mind–body skills and psychotherapy were like the larger logs that kept the fire burning."

However, the plain fact of the matter is that many medications, especially analgesics (pain medicines), seem to work less and less effectively as time goes on. I've seen this in virtually all of my chronic pain patients. Even worse, sometimes certain medications can actually increase the pain. There are several good reasons for this, as we will discuss.

PAIN MEDICATIONS WORK BETTER FOR ACUTE PAIN

Pain of more recent onset is considered acute (duration from immediate to three months). Precisely because it is of more recent origin than chronic pain, it is more amenable to medication treatments. Briefer, more acute pain is less likely to set off chronic muscle bracing and guarding patterns, as well as negative state–dependent memory. Acute pain is far less likely than chronic pain to lead to either central sensitization syndrome (CSS) or autonomic dysregulation (ANS). As a result, pain medications can work more effectively. Once the pain becomes chronic, the interplay of various neurophysiological factors is far more complex, and thus more challenging to treat with medications.

IN CHRONIC PAIN, THE PROBLEM IS
MORE CENTRAL THAN PERIPHERAL

When we charted the life cycle of an acute pain sensation, the signal began at the point of injury, whether that be a toe, a finger, or a low back, and traveled up a peripheral nerve to the central nervous system, where the signal was processed and experienced as pain. The central nervous system does a good job in these cases of generating an accurate signal of the threat that lets you know something is wrong. It also indicates the source of the pain—a nail in the foot, a broken leg, a stomachache.

However, in chronic pain, the problem is not only in the periphery. The problem is also in the central nervous system itself—it is oversensitized and imbalanced. Chronically sensitized nerves result in central system sensitization (CSS) and autonomic dysregulation—a lack of balance between the sympathetic and parasympathetic functions. We can no longer trust the brain's conclusion that a stabbing pain is coming from the back. Its report can be both an exaggeration and a misdirection. It is a lost cause to attempt to treat this centralized pain with medicines designed to treat acute pain in the periphery of the body. You're solving the wrong problem.

This is not to say that there are not still peripheral problems—there are still strained muscles and eroded joints, for example. Rather, an altered central nervous system is complicating things by producing a heightened, distorted report of sensitization and pain.

MEDICATIONS CANNOT CURE CENTRAL
SENSITIZATION OR AUTONOMIC DYSREGULATION

Medications can sometimes be used to suppress the effects of central sensitization and ANS dysregulation. Ill effects of a dysregulated autonomic nervous system can be treated with blood pressure medications, tranquilizers, anticonvulsants, and even some pain medications. Depression from similar kinds of dysregulation can be addressed with antidepressants. But none of these medications get to the root of the problem. Some medications may temporarily put out the brush fire, but can't prevent what is *setting off* the brush fires. Some medications, such as ketamine, have been shown to temporarily reduce central sensitization. However, there are no medications that cure the underlying problem of CSS or ANS dysregulation.

MEDICATION TOLERANCE

Chronic pain sufferers often must take pain medications for longer periods of time. The problem is that often pain medications do not work as well in the long term as they do at first. One reason this happens is that the body builds a tolerance to the medication. When the drug doesn't do its job like it used to, we naturally try a higher dose to see if that works. That works for a while, and so we up the dose again. This becomes especially dangerous when the medication is an opioid, even though medication tolerance is a different problem than addiction. Tolerance may also occur with other types of pain medications, such as non-steroidal anti-inflammatory drugs (NSAIDS), including ibuprofen and naproxen.

MEDICATION INTOLERANCE

Chronic pain sufferers may struggle not only with medication tolerance, but also with medication *intolerance*. Because their central nervous system is sensitized, some patients find that they are not able to tolerate many medications. Many patients that I have treated report that they are so highly sensitive to most medications that it is always very difficult to find a drug they can tolerate sufficiently to gain benefit. The problem of medication intolerance is far more common in chronic than acute pain because the nervous system is more likely to be sensitized.

ANALGESIC REBOUND

Analgesic rebound is what happens when a pain medication starts increasing pain instead of reducing it. We see this bizarre reaction not only in opioids, but also with other types of analgesic pain medications. When rebound occurs, the medications actually aggravate the nerves that carry pain signals. The nerves are altered and sensitized, becoming in themselves an additional pain amplifier. At the same time, the body reacts to rebound by decreasing its secretion of natural painkilling hormones, such as endorphins. This just intensifies the pain. Another problem with rebound is that patients often mistakenly view the rebound effect as a sign that their pain medication has worn off, and therefore they need to just take more of the same drug—which of course sets up a vicious cycle of more pain and more frustration.

MEDICATIONS DON'T TREAT STATE-DEPENDENT MEMORY

A lot of people with chronic pain find that their suffering increases due to negative state–dependent memory. As we discussed earlier, this is the phenomenon where one aspect of a terrible experience will spark a vivid flashback of the entire memory. Like my friend—every time he sees a drill, it makes his finger hurt. Sure, you can reduce some of the intensity of these flashbacks with tranquilizers, antidepressants, and beta–blocking medications, but drugs cannot dismantle the system that brings these bad memories back to us. And medications don't change the suffering caused by a sensitized nervous system combined with traumatic memory. That is the real source of these bouts that alter the intensity and intrusiveness of pain.

MEDICATIONS DON'T REDUCE THE NEGATIVE EMOTIONS ABOUT YOUR CHRONIC PAIN SENSATIONS

Chronic pain is a tough enough problem by itself, but it gets even tougher when people develop secondary reactions to it. A common reaction is bracing and guarding the injured area—which limits mobility and hastens fatigue. Furthermore, the utter frustration of dealing with a pain that won't go away often leads to anxiety and anger. Finally, people get fed up and become unwilling to accept and work with these sensations. In these ways, the presence of the pain sets off an immediate pattern of intolerance or agitation that invariably increases the pain. Antidepressants or tranquilizers may reduce the intensity of this reaction at first, but over time, these secondary reactions make chronic pain much more disruptive.

MEDICATIONS DON'T CORRECT AN ALTERED SENSE OF IDENTITY FROM CHRONIC PAIN

A serious problem that is beyond the reach of medications is that chronic pain patients experience a loss of identity. Their sense of self is altered. I have observed this pattern in many of my patients.

"I used to think of myself as strong, capable, able to respond to problems in resourceful ways," said Cindy, who has chronic abdominal pain. "I used to be proud of my strengths—now I feel as if my very core sense of who I am as a person is permanently diminished." She is a good example of how years of pain have reduced people to feeling like they are being victimized by their own bodies.

OPIOIDS—MULTIPLE TROUBLES FOR CHRONIC PAIN SUFFERERS

I have saved for last what may be the most serious problem in this area— the use of opioid pain medication. Using opioids in the treatment of chronic pain is highly problematic, and it warrants a lengthier discussion. Opioids, also called narcotics, include a range of pharmaceutical preparations often prescribed for pain.

There is no doubt that opioids can sometimes be helpful for acute and severe pain. They are sometimes helpful in the treatment of pain related to a terminal illness, such as later stage cancer pain. However, there is increasing data showing that many cancer patients now suffer with opioid addition.

The United States consumes 83 percent of the world's opioids. Yet, there is no evidence that they are helpful in chronic pain. Up to 40,000 people die every year due to opioids, and most of these started because of chronic pain.

In most cases, it all begins when a well-meaning prescriber recommends opioids to help patients deal with acute pain. Frequently, the patient is in pain due to an injury, a surgery, or even just a tooth extraction. If you are taking opioids, rest assured that nobody is blaming you or judging you for having gotten on them.

The opioid crisis emerged in the late 1990s, when opioid pain medications were prescribed at greater and greater rates. The pharmaceutical companies that made the opioid medications told providers that their patients would not become addicted. This turned out to be misinformation. It soon became apparent that opioids were highly addictive. The National Institute for Drug Abuse estimates that, by 2017, more than 47,000 Americans had died as a result of opioid overdose. Another 1.7 million Americans suffered from substance use disorders related to prescription opioid pain medications. It is now clear that prescription opioids carry significant risks, and they often lead to serious side effects.

Common types of opioid narcotics

- OxyContin (oxycodone)
- Vicodin (hydrocodone)
- Morphine
- Heroin
- Synthetic opioids
  - Fentanyl (fifty times stronger than heroin; a hundred times stronger than morphine). Note: most cases of fentanyl-related overdose and death are linked to the rise in illegally made fentanyl, sold through illegal drug markets due to its heroin-like effects (source: CDC)
  - Methadone
  - Tramadol

Anyone taking prescription opioids can become addicted and is at risk for accidental overdose, or even death. According to the American Medical Association, about 45 percent of heroin users started with an addiction to prescription opioids.

The risks of opioids are so great profound that a new category of addiction known as Opioid Use Disorder (OUD) has been recognized by the American Psychiatric Association. OUD has been included in the latest version of the *Diagnostic and Statistical Manual of Mental Disorders, Fifth Edition* (DSM–5). It describes OUD as a problematic pattern of opioid use leading to distress. The problems related to OUD include:

- Spending a great deal of time recovering from the effects of opioids

- Problems fulfilling obligations at work, home, and school

- Reducing or giving up activities due to opioid use

- Taking larger amounts of the drug

- Taking opioids over a longer period than prescribed

- Experiencing withdrawal

- Taking opioids to reduce withdrawal symptoms

Even when taken as directed, the use of prescription opioids can cause several side effects. Among them is a condition called "opioid–induced hyperalgesia." Hyperalgesia means an abnormally heightened sensitivity to pain. There is evidence that opioid medications cause sensitization of the central nervous system even after a short period of use. When this occurs, the very drug used to reduce pain will actually increase the pain.

When opioids lead to physical dependence because of the pain, addiction often follows. That's because opioids also affect parts of the brain that mediate pleasure and reward. The craving for that pleasure may exceed the drug's ability to relieve pain. That's when addiction arises, which gives the patient a new problem to face in addition to the chronic pain problem. This sort of addiction tends to come more easily to a person with a preexisting problem with chemical dependency or substance abuse. Whether it is dependency on alcohol, tranquilizers, or another substance—that person is at higher risk for opioid addiction.

Aside from addiction, opiate use has a host of possible side effects that can be very problematic. A person may suffer from nausea and vomiting, dizziness, sedation, drowsiness, confusion, and problems with judgement and decision—making. Opioids can cause balance problems and increase the risk of falls—especially in the elderly. They can disturb sleep quality. Digestion can get slowed, leading to opioid—induced constipation, or OIC. Severe OIC is so common that other medications are needed to counteract it, often leading to further digestive symptoms. And since withdrawal symptoms are so severe, it may create significant motivation to continue using opioids to prevent them.

HOW OPIATES INTERFERE WITH REHABILITATION

Chronic pain patients who take opiates have greater challenges than chronic pain sufferers who do not take opiates. For one thing, opiates often intensify the pain by causing central sensitization. Their pain has also likely been made greater by analgesic rebound, where the medication itself increases their pain. This person is likely drowsy and exhausted due to the sedating effects of opiates and because opiates disturb their sleep cycle. They are far more likely to be constipated from the opiates. Plus, constipation leads to digestive pain, cramping, bloating, and distention.

One of the biggest problems with opiates is that they work through dissociation. They disconnect the person from awareness of sensations and emotions occurring in the body. This may be helpful for acute pain. However, over time, dissociation from one's body and emotions interferes with the healing process. Opioid—enhanced dissociation essentially undercuts the entire rehabilitation process. My approach to tackling chronic pain is founded upon developing awareness of your body and your emotions. Awareness is the A of the ABC method. Opiates alter and distort the patient's relationship to the sensations and emotions of the body.

Strong negative emotions are a normal part of the process of coping with chronic pain. The sense that your body has betrayed you leads to feelings of anger, frustration, grief, despair, resentment, even shame and disgust. These are difficult feelings to deal with. Nevertheless, you must deal with them to heal, and dealing effectively with your difficult emotions will lead to further improvements. And when you are disconnected from your emotions by the effects of opioid use, this interferes with your healing from chronic pain.

Think of addiction as being driven by any substance or activity that helps you to avoid unpleasant feelings or experiences. Opioids not only dissociate you from painful sensations in your back; they also numb away the experience of these painful emotions. This powerful force of emotional addiction just adds to the big issue of physical addiction. It's a double threat. This twin addiction becomes reinforced every time the opioids unplug you from the sensations and emotions of your body.

Another hazard of opioid addiction is the "phobic" feelings one has toward bodily sensations. As you may guess, this fearful attitude reinforces the nervous system's "false alarms" that plague the chronic pain sufferer. Patients on opioids often react with fear, annoyance, and bracing to even nonthreatening sensations. To prevent these sensations from being interpreted as threats by the limbic system—which sets off the fight–flight response—the patient needs to learn different strategies for self–soothing. This will subdue the challenges of painful sensations, and will promote healing.

We will review how to change this pattern in the "Cultivating" section of this book, specifically when I teach you about Limbic Retraining.

When I treat a patient who has been on opioids, I know they are struggling with all the problems discussed above. They have become increasingly estranged from their body, and from all the natural internal mechanisms that we possess for self-soothing. This can be turned around. But first the patient needs to understand how the opioids have affected them and have unwittingly interfered with their rehabilitation. To rehabilitate well, the chronic pain sufferer needs to be able to connect with sensations in their body. They must learn to respond to bodily cues differently before more pain occurs.

CONSIDERATIONS FOR PATIENTS CONSIDERING OPIOID USE

Given all the risks associated with opioids, you should not consider using them without first having a detailed discussion with your health provider. Together you should look at the pros and cons. Will the benefits of prescription opioids outweigh their many possible dangers? If you begin opioid treatment and your pain is not resolving as quickly as expected, you should follow up promptly with your health provider. You should expect that urine testing will be conducted during the course of your therapy.

Before you start your opioid regimen, you should think ahead and plan the endgame. Once it is time to stop opioid treatment, you need instructions on how to taper down safely to minimize withdrawal symptoms. Most importantly, your approach to healing from chronic pain should include a good mix of non-opioid treatment modalities. As I always say to my patients, "If you're going to take something away, you need to replace it with something else." It is never a good idea to rely on narcotics without also practicing a range of healthy self-care activities. These will include regular stretching exercises, physical exercise such as walking, calming exercises, and self-hypnosis. You need to create a balance between activity and rest in your daily schedule. Proper nutrition is important, along with establishing the proper amount of social interaction and support.

MEDICATIONS FOR CHRONIC PAIN: CONCLUSION

With all the concerns discussed above, are there appropriate uses for medications to help in healing from chronic pain? Yes, but only if the drugs are used as a bridge to feel a different experiential state, and if you are learning vital self-care and self-healing skills at the same time. Medications for chronic pain can be helpful for interrupting a cycle of pain. This also disrupts ongoing patterns of negative neuroplasticity, so you can start anew. Just keep in mind that "brief usage" is the key phrase setting a limit on such medications. The actual length of time that you stay on your medication will vary, depending on whether it is an analgesic pain reliever, minor tranquilizer, anticonvulsant, muscle relaxant, or antidepressant medication. Obviously, this will be determined through thoughtful discussion with your prescriber and healing team.

It is very important to work with a prescriber who understands this balance between medication and self-care skills. In this context, the two of you can specify what you expect your medications to achieve—as well as what they cannot achieve.

An appropriate plan for using the drug would look something like this: "I will take just enough pain medication to take the edge off certain episodes of back pain so that I can get up and walk six blocks as part of my self-care."

An inappropriate drug use plan would be like this: "I will take enough pain medication to no longer have to care that my pain is there. I want to 'check out' and not have to do anything else to manage it."

This second plan is a bad idea, because it is likely to lead to much greater frustration and dissatisfaction with the medication.

In conclusion, even if opioids didn't carry all the dangers and side effects they do, I would generally caution against their use because of all the ways I've listed above that narcotics interfere with rehabilitation and healing.

In the following sections of the book, I will discuss many non-pharmaceutical strategies that work more effectively for chronic pain and with far fewer side effects.

SECTION II

Setting the Stage

Introduction to Setting the Stage

After suffering for months and years with chronic pain, you are only too familiar with how the experience feels like a dreary, intense, exhausting, never-ending journey. Striving to cope with the daily demands of chronic pain feels like struggling to stay on a path that is treacherous. Trying to find relief is like being on a road that is rocky, winding, and confusing. It can feel like you're lost, wandering through thick woods, reaching many dead ends along the way.

What you need is a map, a new guide, to reorient yourself to the path from suffering and hopelessness to healing. You need to change direction, to put your life on a new track. You need trail signs along the way to help you stay on the path when you occasionally, inevitably, lose your way. And along the way, discovering that hope and healing are possible, even after years of reaching endless dead ends.

For over thirty-six years, I have been guiding chronic pain patients on their healing journey. Over this time, I have discovered where the dead ends are, where the roadblocks and obstacles are hidden. I have learned which paths lead to the healing destination, and I want to make sure you are well-prepared as you embark on your journey. Just as you would stockpile supplies for a long hiking trip—a good backpack, nourishing food, plenty of water, a first-aid kit, accurate maps and GPS, and of course a skilled trail guide to lead you safely to your destination—I want you to be well-prepared as you embark.

The purpose of this section of the book is to make sure you are well-prepared before you embark on your treatment. Getting a good start will maximize your chances for success.

You need to consider these five items as you prepare to get started:

1. Determine your current stage on the healing journey.

2. Select the types of professionals who will be most helpful in your treatment.

3. Understand—and embrace—the crucial importance of self-care in healing from chronic pain.

4. Fill out your own personal pain assessment, just as if I was taking your history in person in my office.

5. Know the path and trajectory of the healing journey, to be prepared for the inevitable ups and downs while staying the course.

CHAPTER 7

Where Are You on the Healing Journey: Diagnostic Phase or Rehabilitation Phase?

As I have already mentioned, you need to have a diagnosis for your chronic pain condition before you are ready for this book. But here is a very important question: Do you trust your diagnosis? Your answer may affect how you go about making your problem better. The way you view your condition will determine your choice of treatments, as well as your commitment to practices for taking care of yourself. After all, for many acute problems, little or no self-care is needed. Break your leg? Get a cast for a few weeks and it's fixed. Strep throat? Take your antibiotics for ten days and you should be good to go.

We've learned that, with chronic problems, it's not so simple. There is usually no magic bullet for chronic pain. No medication or surgical intervention can fix the problem. In the pain medicine field, we use the terms *diagnostic phase* and *rehabilitation phase* to describe where patients are on their healing trajectory.

DIAGNOSTIC PHASE

If you have chronic pain or live with a chronic pain sufferer, you are likely very familiar with the diagnostic phase. This is where you go to x number of clinics, hospitals, and specialists, trying to find out what is wrong. Your search for a diagnosis may entail physical examinations, blood tests, X-rays, CT or MRI scans, or diagnostic nerve blocks. If these tests reveal a specific structural or biomechanical problem to explain your current symptoms, then the diagnosis will call for a prescribed treatment. You may find that surgery, nerve blocks, or steroid or biologic immune-modulating medications will help your symptoms improve.

However, in the case of many chronic conditions, symptoms persist and worsen even after these diagnoses are made. Your current symptoms may persist or even get worse after the initial physical problem has been repaired. I've had patients who have had surgery to successfully repair herniated lumbar discs, yet their low back pain continued for years. Some patients just can't stop looking for that magic bullet that they hope will take the problem away, and keep getting referred to more and more specialists.

REHABILITATION PHASE

Fortunately, some patients get referred to a pain clinic, where the specialists are more highly trained in how chronic conditions differ from acute ones. Once a diagnosis is clarified and confirmed, the clinician will educate the patient on the need to move on from the diagnostic phase to the *rehabilitation* phase. This is a necessary step in the journey of healing from chronic pain.

In this phase, you know what your diagnosis is, and you accept it. You become committed to following a course of *slow, steady, progressive progress* in your symptoms. You no longer demand that the pain disappear completely. Instead, you adopt a more realistic goal of reducing the frequency, intensity, and intrusiveness of the pain. This reduction in pain allows you to get back to your desired activities of daily living. You have started the process of developing your own internal toolkit for healing, without depending on an external "rescue" treatment.

Over the years, I have encountered many patients with chronic pain who were not quite ready to make the transition from diagnostic to rehabilitation phase. This is the person who clings to the hope that a physical cause for their pain just hasn't been found yet. There might still be "something missing that a third MRI might reveal." "Maybe there's a tumor or a growth on my spine that remains hidden." "Maybe I have some rare autoimmune condition causing my pain that hasn't shown up on blood tests yet." These holdouts will have trouble truly committing themselves to the sustained effort, or enjoying the benefits, of self-care. After all, why should they bother doing stretching exercises every day if their whole problem might be solved by another surgery?

TIMING IS EVERYTHING

When I meet a new patient who clearly is not ready for the rehabilitation phase, I always tell them the same thing:

"I realize that you still have the belief and hope that another diagnostic evaluation and MRI will reveal a new, specific cause for your chronic pain. From my reading of your chart and discussions with your other providers, I do not feel that additional diagnostic evaluation is needed. However, if this is your belief, then I support you to go through the additional time, expense, and effort needed to get yet another evaluation. If a new treatable diagnosis is discovered that leads to better treatments for you, that would be great. But if it doesn't lead to new diagnoses and conclusions, I want to remind you to not be discouraged. There is another course of action, healing, and rehabilitation available for you here, when you are ready for it."

CHAPTER 8
Your Healing Team

From our earlier discussion you learned how chronic pain is like the old story of the Six Blind Men and the Elephant. There are many different aspects to chronic pain, and they must be treated in a unified fashion. This is why you benefit from a team of providers skilled in chronic pain and its treatment. They each see the same problem from slightly different perspectives.

So what kinds of healthcare professionals should be on your healing team?

Most people have a primary care physician for their general health needs. This clinician most often would be an internist or a family practitioner. Occasionally, some women may choose to see their gynecologist (OB–GYN) for their primary care needs. This is useful and appropriate for most general health concerns, particularly when the problem is acute, of recent onset. This is the place to address everyday health problems and ongoing health maintenance. This is the place for annual physical examinations, cuts, broken bones, infections, recent–onset headache, recent–onset back pain, digestive distress, and so on.

However, as you have read here so far, chronic pain lasting longer than three to six months is more complex to treat. There are multiple factors affecting your pain beyond the physical realm, and into emotional, social, recreational, vocational, financial, and legal spheres as well. Research tells us that a multidisciplinary team is the most effective way of treating chronic pain. Because of the complexity of chronic pain, no single specialist has the expertise to assess and manage it independently. The goal of multidisciplinary pain treatment is not only to provide good pain relief, but also to improve physical, psychological, and behavioral functioning.

YOU ARE NOT STARTING FROM SCRATCH

If the notion of assembling a healing team seems like a daunting or even impossible task, not to worry. You are not starting from scratch here. Most likely, you are already being treated by your primary care physician, and possibly also an additional physician pain specialist such as a neurologist or orthopedist. You can proceed right now, confidently, using the ABC method. My goal in educating you about the healing team is to empower you on your healing journey by supplementing your healing team with a few additional highly skilled health professionals to help you on your way.

Advancement on the chronic pain journey can feel arduous, frustrating, and sometimes downright impossible! Since chronic pain has multiple causes, you need to be provided with education, skills, and training in how to deal well with relapses. Having the skilled guidance and reassurance of a team of specialized practitioners provides the foundation of support needed to achieve successful healing.

Some people might be able to find these services through an integrated chronic pain treatment program in a hospital or outpatient clinic. These programs house all the professionals you need to see in one place. However, there are a decreasing number of accredited multidisciplinary chronic pain programs in the United States. An increasingly common scenario is for chronic pain patients to form their own team. They find providers in the community who can work together, even though they are not located in the same clinic.

ASSEMBLING YOUR HEALING TEAM

Your healing team is a group of health professionals who will help you to maximize your quality of life. At a minimum, your team should include:

- **Your primary care physician.**

- **Another physician** who has specialized experience treating chronic pain, such as a neurologist, rheumatologist (specializing in diseases of joints, muscles, and surrounding soft tissue), or physiatrist (a.k.a. a physical medicine and rehabilitation specialist).

- **A physical therapist (PT)**—Be sure to find one with specialized training and experience in treating various types of chronic pain. The PT may provide massage and manipulation of joints and muscles. They may advise on posture and exercises to relieve pain, and may use such treatments as heat, ultrasound, and traction to improve pain symptoms.

- **A clinical psychologist** with specialized training in assessment and treatment of chronic pain. This PhD-level clinician should be trained and experienced in the multitude of physical and psychological factors that can affect your pain. The psychologist helps reduce emotional distress associated with chronic pain and helps the patient develop skills to help cope with stress and pain.

Additional providers may also be helpful, including nurses, social workers, and occupational therapists. Dentists who treat head and neck pain (such as temporomandibular disorders, or TMJ) may also be beneficial collaborators.

Everyone on your team should be conversant in the core concepts of pain medicine, including central sensitization, autonomic dysregulation, and the importance of addressing any complicating factors such as depression, anxiety, or trauma.

THINGS TO KEEP IN MIND
WITH YOUR TEAM

There are certain standards to follow, whether you seek out an integrated team program affiliated with a hospital or health plan (a "one-stop-shop"), or individual providers who treat chronic pain.

TEAM COMMUNICATION

All the members of your healing team should have experience in treating chronic pain and be willing to collaborate with each other. They need to know about the others and keep open lines of communication. Successful chronic pain treatment requires continuity of care, where all the team members are operating from the same playbook. Each of them should remain open to ideas from other team members—even if they might not agree with them. They should offer suggestions and treatments that are consistent with the rest of the team. If one or more of the team members give suggestions that are inconsistent or contradictory with the rest of the team, you need to have your team correct this problem.

The various clinicians should be receptive to discussing your care with them, and should not make you feel rushed during your treatment session. They should be prepared to admit when the answer to your question is not known, and should show willingness to do some additional digging to find out what they don't know. Furthermore, they should be willing to communicate with your family as well.

BE YOUR OWN BEST ADVOCATE

The most important member of your healing team is *you*. The more you actively participate in the process, the better the outcomes will be. Be sure to ask questions when you are unclear about the various types of treatments and exercises they recommend. If you are wondering about how a particular treatment or exercise fits in to your overall healing goals, ask about it. The more you know about these details, the more likely you will be to follow through consistently with all suggestions. (Read more about your responsibilities in the next section, "The Role of Self-Care in Healing from Chronic Pain.")

It feels very reassuring to have a team of great health practitioners supporting your healing journey. If you need help finding clinicians in your area who can provide these services, these resources may be helpful:

- International Association for the Study of Pain

- National Fibromyalgia & Chronic Pain Association

- American Academy of Pain Medicine

CHAPTER 9

The Role of Self-Care in Healing from Chronic Pain

"Self-care is the foundation of successful chronic pain treatment."

—Dr. Daniel Clauw, University of Michigan Pain Treatment Program

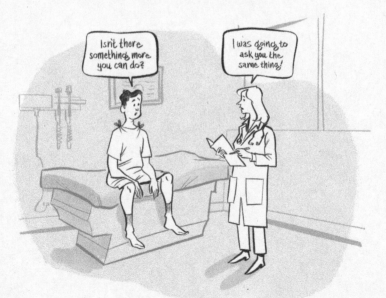

Several years ago, I attended the annual meeting of the National Academy of Medicine. They discussed the state of the healthcare system in the United States. One speaker after another emphasized the US system's excellence, among the best in the world, for treating acute illness. For Whether treating heart disease, stroke, or cancer, Western biomedicine is second to none. However, we are far less successful when it comes to treating chronic illnesses. We have a lot to learn when it comes to treating chronic pain, respiratory diseases, asthma, hypertension, chronic kidney disease, and diabetes.

Why this big disparity between treating acute illnesses and chronic diseases? They concluded that part of the reason is that, for acute problems, all the treatments are delivered by the practitioners. The patients don't have to do anything except take their medications or show up for surgery. There is usually a good result from prescribing an antibiotic for strep throat, resetting a broken bone, or surgically removing a tumor. However, in the case of a chronic illness, medications and surgical techniques are not enough. For healing to occur for chronic conditions, patients need to be active participants in their own care. Self-care behaviors include such things as eating a healthy diet, having social interaction, and getting regular exercise. The patient needs to allow themself to rest without feeling guilty. They need to become adept at monitoring their symptoms. The conference concluded that, for us to achieve better outcomes in treatment of chronic conditions, health professionals need to do a better job of motivating their patients to get actively involved in their own self-care.

WHY ARE SELF-CARE STRATEGIES SO IMPORTANT?

If chronic pain is not effectively treated, it can beget further problems that ultimately worsen it. That is the finding of several multidisciplinary pain treatment programs, such as the one at the University of Michigan. Chronic pain can cause more stress, less activity, poorer sleep, obesity, and illness behaviors—such as clenching muscles or overexerting when feeling better. These problems become bigger issues over time, and can cause central sensitization to worsen. It should be noted that none of these problems can be treated with medication. *However, good sleep, relaxation skills, and proper physical exercises can activate the most powerful pain-relieving systems in the body.* This self-care approach, supported over time, is the most effective treatment for these problems.

CHALLENGES TO MAINTAINING A SELF-CARE ROUTINE

Progress in chronic pain depends on the patient's willingness to participate actively in their self-care. Nevertheless, patients have difficulty maintaining self-care routines for various reasons.

In my experience, the first signs of difficulty with self-care usually appear in the second appointment. This is when the patient comes back and reports on their first efforts at self-care. They tell me what progress they have made on strategies they learned in the first appointment—such as a simple breathing technique, monitoring their pain intensity during the day, and noticing their posture. Invariably, at this second appointment, the patient and I discuss the various challenges and obstacles interfering with their self-care practice.

Part of the challenge in healing from chronic pain is that it's not like just "flipping a switch" and then having it change. Rather, it's a process, occurring over time. The analogy I often use for describing the process of chronic pain rehabilitation is swimming in the ocean. If you are swimming in the ocean, you might effectively swim a strong hundred yards. But when you turn your head to the side to check your progress, all you see is more water! It's as if nothing at all has changed. And if you feel like nothing has changed after lots of repetition and hard work, you're certainly not inclined to invest more time and effort. This is why noticing and acknowledging small improvements is so important. More on this later.

Some patients don't have support for their self-care from family or friends. They may have a spouse or family member who doesn't understand their need for self-care time and then becomes unhappy or disgruntled. They may not follow through on these tasks due to depression or anxiety. They may feel discouraged if their pain relief strategies don't seem to be working well. They may feel they don't have time to do self-care because of time constraints and other priorities. Or they may avoid exercise or other self-care activity out of a fear of worsening their pain.

Sometimes pain sufferers don't do self-care because of faulty underlying beliefs. Some may believe that, if their pain is helped by their self-care, that this means, "If you still have chronic pain, then it's your fault for not doing self-care, or not doing it well enough."

For those who think this way, we address the issue further. I clarify that their chronic pain is not their fault, even when doing self-care helps. What I further illuminate is how the patient can empower themselves to have more positive impact over their pain. I remind them, "It's not about this being your *fault*, because it isn't. But if there is the possibility that you can have more *impact* on your pain, would you like to see that happen?" Virtually every patient eagerly answers "Yes" to that question.

Some are concerned that, if their pain is improved by these exercises, then, "Maybe I don't have 'real' biological illness causing my pain." So many chronic pain patients have been through an exhaustive series of tests and procedures, only to be told that there is no good reason for their pain, or else that nothing more can be done. For many sufferers, the phrase "biological illness" is code-language for "My pain is real!" The patient gets caught in a double bind: they either do some self-care, but fear that their pain will be exposed as being "fake" or "not biological," or they hesitate to do the very self-care activities that would actually provide the most help!

My message to such sufferers is always the same: your pain is absolutely real. And, like the rest of our life experience, everything that we feel and sense has a biological component to it. The crux of the issue is that the real biological problem occurring may not be only a herniated disc, but also an altered central nervous system. Once this is understood, we can move ahead toward a healing plan. As this is understood, you will start to naturally feel more motivated to avail yourself of the help and healing that come from regular practice of walking, calming techniques, stretching, and quieting an agitated mind.

I also find that, when someone does not follow through on recommendations for self-care activities, there are other common reasons for this. Some don't believe that the self-care activity (for example, a stretching or breathing technique) will help their pain. Others tend to prioritize their own needs as less important than the needs and demands of others around them, so there is no time and energy left by day's end for caring for self.

We will need to explore whether you have difficulty feeling entitled to attend to your own needs while others need something from you. I'm reminded about when I am on an airplane, taxiing toward the runway for takeoff. The flight attendant, as part of their pre-flight instructions, says, "In the event of loss of cabin pressure, be sure to secure your own oxygen mask before helping others." Of course this makes sense, as you will be more able to help someone else if you are first able to breathe yourself! This story applies well to self-care in general. The better you take care of yourself, the more you will be capable and available to respond to others' needs.

Jake, a patient of mine in his early eighties, was seeing me for treatment of chronic pain in his middle and lower back. He was also tending to his wife, who was suffering from multiple health conditions including hip pain, knee pain, headaches, fatigue, and diabetes. His wife's ailments were Jake's central focus, taking up much of the day with massaging her, reading to her, and driving her to medical appointments. Jake would usually postpone any of his self-care activities (walking, breathing techniques, self-hypnosis, socializing with friends) until he was assured that he had taken care of everything for his wife. And, as you might imagine, his exhaustion at the end of the day left little room for attention to self. Not surprisingly, his own pain symptoms were getting gradually more severe. Being very bright, Jake intellectually knew all the reasons why he needed to do the self-care. This didn't lead to him practicing regularly, however. At least not until I pointed out to him: "Did it ever occur to you that the biggest reason you need to make time for your self-care is so that you can feel well enough to continue to be present for your wife and feel well enough to respond to her needs?" This brought the issue home to him, and helped him to finally find the motivation to commit to regular self-care. Not only did it reduce his pain, but his wife was quite relieved to see that her Jake was feeling better!

We may need to look at how you learned to believe that your needs are less important than others'. Were you taught that focusing on yourself is selfish? Do you feel guilt when you take time for yourself?

Once we have identified the obstacle(s) to your regular self-care practice, we can begin formulating a plan for a course correction. Maybe we need to discuss whether you actually believe that a particular exercise or stretching technique will help you. Here is a strategy I use with my patients when this occurs. In my office, I will ask you to rate your level of discomfort on a 0   10 scale. Then I will ask you to do the exercise in my office (for example, a brief breathing technique). Then I will ask you once again to rate the discomfort level. Almost always, the pain level has decreased. This provides some experiential and empirical proof that it works.

So, the next step in your plan is to aim for small, measurable changes in self-care. For example, start by committing to practice just one self-care activity, a certain number of times daily (for example, a 4-4-8 breathing technique for three minutes, three times a day, for three days). And when you accomplish this, acknowledge it! Give yourself some acknowledgement, and perhaps a small reward—something that is enjoyable for you, and hopefully healthy. Buy some flowers or plants for your garden. Go hear a music performance. Celebrating these small incremental steps provides encouragement for keeping up the good work, and serves as a reminder that you are in fact making progress.

FOUR IMPORTANT KEYS TO MAINTAINING SUCCESSFUL SELF-CARE

1. Pay very close attention to even small improvements in your symptoms.

2. Reward yourself for these small improvements.

3. Keep practicing.

4. Build resilience.

You will find valuable examples of these four keys in the final section of this book, "Conclusion: Maintain Your Gains Now and In the Future."

CHAPTER 10

Your Personal Pain Assessment

It is often said, "Assessment is the beginning of treatment." Very well, let's begin. I want to take you through an assessment of your particular pain problem, as if you were my patient sitting across from me in my office. My hope and intention is that, as you read and consider these questions, it will open the door to greater understanding of the factors affecting your pain. As you have learned so far, chronic pain is a complex problem. Accordingly, an assessment of all the psychophysiological factors affecting your pain must be broad and multifaceted. The questions themselves will inform you of what issues are important for a successful treatment.

Even as I present my questions, you are probably already asking yourself one: "Why do I need to see a psychologist?" You may even have a question for me: "Do you think my problems are all in my head?"

I will start by explaining why you are seeing a clinical health psychologist for your pain problem. In answer to your question of me, "No, I don't think your chronic pain is all in your head." The idea that such a problem is psychosomatic betrays a misunderstanding about chronic pain. It also follows an outdated logic that assumes the mind and body are distinct from each other. Since your diagnosis affirms there is no active physical disease accounting for your pain, the only choice remaining is that it must be psychosomatic. The problem, however, is that most patients with complex chronic pain fall between the cracks of this false dichotomy.

We now know, thanks to advanced brain imaging and research findings from the field of psychoneuroimmunology, that our thoughts, emotions, and bodies are totally interconnected via neurophysiological and hormonal processes. Chronic pain represents a complex synergy of physical and psychological factors interacting through our brain and nervous system. The complexity of chronic pain requires an approach that combines the intricacies of psychophysiology. That's where a clinical health psychologist comes in.

A clinical health psychologist possesses a doctoral degree in clinical psychology, followed by advanced specialty training or a fellowship in neurophysiology, learning, memory, perception, cognition, and motivation. Their specialty training takes place in settings that treat chronic health problems, such as chronic pain, orthopedics, neurological rehabilitation, and cardiology, as well as in primary care settings such as internal medicine and pediatrics. They are specialists in understanding and treating how physical and psychological factors interact in chronic illnesses, such as chronic pain. This is why you were referred to a clinical health psychologist for your pain problem.

Now to the assessment. In the lines below each question, please write down your response.

Please describe the pain problems that bring you in today.

For example, "I suffer from chronic low back pain that radiates down my left leg. I also have problems with fatigue and poor sleep."

_____

_____

_____

_____

_____

_____

_____

_____

_____

_____

_____

_____

_____

When did the symptoms first begin? Did they begin with a precipitating event or did it come on gradually?

For example, "My back pain began after a period of heavy lifting at my warehouse job over ten years ago. I have had multiple evaluations and tests and there are no slipped or bulging discs in my back. The pain has persisted since then and has gradually increased in intensity."

How does your pain present? Is it constant or intermittent? Do you notice fluctuations in the pain, or does it seem more constant to you?

The experience of your chronic pain may be like a constant, heavy weight that you carry all day, every day, leaving you exhausted by the burden. For some, the pain exhibits a predictable pattern, perhaps being fairly mild in the morning, then increasing gradually during the day and looming as a major hindrance by dinner time. For others it is exactly the opposite: pain wakes them in the morning because it's so severe, and then gradually decreases as they get involved in the tasks of the day. And for others, the pain is so frustrating precisely because it shows no detectable pattern. Sometimes it's worse in the morning, sometimes in the evening, or mid-day—a seemingly random cycle of occurrence. For some people, the random occurrence of pain leads them to feel increasingly victimized and powerless.

Does the pain occur in just one area or does it spread to different areas?

For some people, the pain is focused in one location, perhaps in the back of their head or in the center of their low back. For others, the pain may start in the lower back, but then radiate down their leg. Fibromyalgia sufferers may describe widespread pain in their neck, shoulders, legs, and arms.

What terms do you use to describe your pain?

Which of the following terms describe your pain: sharp, dull, aching, burning, stabbing, pressure, knife-like, gnawing, heavy, shooting, sickening, throbbing, tiring, cramping? This is just a partial list that may not include how you would describe the pain. These descriptors are very important to the healing process. For one thing, they convey the personal impact of your unique pain. They also provide hints about what physical mechanisms may be at work (such as neuropathic pain, myofascial pain, etc.).

How do you rate the intensity of your pain right now on a 0–10 scale? [Where 0 is no pain and 10 is the worst pain that you have ever experienced in your life]

I get a lot of complaints at first about using the 0 – 10 pain rating scale. "Oh, I hate doing those. They're so useless." Actually, they're not useless. It is an important and helpful tool for multiple reasons. First, it is an immediate way to help patients to be more active in their self-care. That is a top priority, according to a 2012 Institute of Medicine report entitled, "Living Well with Chronic Illness: A Call for Public Health Action." The scale also improves self-monitoring skills. It's important for sufferers to notice the daily fluctuations in the intensity of pain. It is also useful in finding out whether the patient is able to observe these fluctuations, or is too numb to sense the difference, or is exaggerating.

The scale is also a useful way to determine whether the exercises and other self-care activities are actually helping or not by measuring before and after. Plus, the scale can be used for more than just pain; patients can report on their levels of intrusiveness, tension, hopelessness, and other variables. The scale can even be used to measure the patient's level of interest in maintaining self-care.

The scale is also a way to measure progress on the long journey of self-healing. It's like swimming in the ocean. You may go a hundred yards, but you look around and it all seems the same. It's hard to gauge the progress you have already made. Having ways to measure small changes makes the journey manageable and gives a realistic sense of advancement.

(Pain intensity right now on 0–10 scale)

_____

_____

_____

_____

Can you discern differences in your pain level throughout the day?

Research suggests that most chronic pain patients are able to notice differences in pain intensity throughout the day. They tend to say that it feels worse later in the day, that it feels better after a massage and feels worse when the barometric pressure changes. A smaller percentage of patients report no fluctuation in pain levels throughout the day. This means one of two things. One, they may be one of those rare individuals whose pain never changes intensity. Or two, they have difficulty noticing their bodily sensations closely enough to be aware of any change in intensity. This is likely due to a coping strategy called dissociation, in which the sufferer has learned to ignore the pain by focusing their attention elsewhere. By distracting their awareness from the pain, they are better able to make it through the day. If this is your experience, let me reassure you that there are safe, gentle, and effective ways to build this useful skill of somatic awareness—paying attention to bodily sensations.

(Can you discern differences in pain level throughout the day? Y / N)

Triggers: What do you find increases the pain?

Do these things increase your pain? Bending, lifting, standing for a long time, barometric pressure changes, fatigue, poor sleep, different kinds of stress (either external stresses, such as financial problems, a difficult boss, or marital conflict; or internal stresses, such as depression, anxiety, worry, etc.), caffeine, sugar, foods with gluten, etc.

_____

_____

_____

_____

_____

_____

_____

_____

_____

_____

_____

_____

What do you find decreases the pain?

This may include variables such as rest, mild exercise, breathing techniques, stretching, self-hypnosis, ibuprofen, heat, or cold.

If you can't name anything that decreases the pain—is it because you haven't been successful at finding any relief? Or is it because you have difficulty sensing changes in how your body feels? Your answer could reflect your longstanding frustration and hopelessness that absolutely nothing can reduce your pain.

As your treatment progresses, you will become aware of many additional factors—those that make the pain worse, as well as things that decrease the pain. You can use this information to make yourself feel better.

Does stress affect your pain? If so, what sorts of things do you find to be most stressful? [People often have highly individual notions of stress.]

Stress is a broad term that is widely interpreted. People use the word in many ways. You might think that, since it applies to everything, it doesn't mean anything.

Nothing could be further from the truth. Research reveals that stress activates certain physiological processes, and that it has a definite effect on pain. Allow me to offer a definition: "Stress is the perception that your capacity to cope has been exceeded."

Some patients are afraid to admit that stress impacts their pain, because they think it means it is psychosomatic. They end up saying that stress does not affect their pain. In my experience, it is far more common that a patient will say stress does affect their pain. Once you understand the physiology of pain and stress, you realize that it is an inescapable fact that stress affects pain. And so, if a patient says, "Stress isn't a factor," my interest will be piqued as to why this is the case. As part of the follow-up on this, I will review the physiology of stress and remark that it would be quite unusual for stress *not* to affect their pain.

(In what ways do you find that stress affects your pain?)

What treatments have been attempted for this problem? Have they been helpful? If not, why do you think these treatments haven't worked? What do *you* think is causing your symptoms?

When your pain has lasted for a very long time, has anyone asked your opinion about why the pain persists despite all efforts to reduce it? Sometimes your response can provide a valuable insight. You might think of something that nobody else has thought of before.

Do you have other physical illnesses or symptoms?

Very often, patients with chronic pain may have other physical conditions affecting their health. Some have heart disease, which may affect their ability to do regular exercise. Some may have diabetes, which could cause a type of pain called *diabetic neuropathy*. This causes sensations of tingling, burning, or numbness in your hands and feet. Some patients may have conditions such as Lupus, Crohn's disease, or Multiple Sclerosis. If you have one of these autoimmune disorders, your immune system may mistakenly attack healthy tissues in your body. You may then need to take powerful medications such as steroids, which reduce inflammation but may cause you to feel tense or agitated. I assume that you and your primary care physician have implemented plans of action for these problems. We need to discuss these other conditions to ensure we understand your pain from every possible angle.

Do you have a primary care physician? Who are the other health professionals that you currently see?

To take part in the ABC program of healing from chronic pain, you need a complete medical evaluation from your primary care provider or other specialist. You must ensure that any and all organic health problems have been diagnosed and treated. Also, as we discussed above, effective treatment of chronic pain requires a team approach. It is vitally important that you maintain good communication with all members of your team. This team includes your primary care physician, a physical therapist, a clinical psychologist, and other clinicians that you see regularly. These may include nurse practitioners, physician assistants, craniosacral therapists, nutritionists, or others. A collaborative team will provide good continuity of care going forward. You ought not to be stressed and needlessly confused by being given competing diagnoses from different practitioners.

What medications are you currently taking? What medications
were you taking previously? Are your medications prescribed
by one or multiple prescribers? How long have you been on
_____ medication? [asked for each medication:] How is
this medication working for you? What is your expectation
for this medication? Is that occurring? [Checking to see if
expectations are realistic]

This question can open a discussion about the role of medications in
an integrative healing approach. Patients may also have misleading
expectations regarding meds. Multiple prescribers can be an issue,
especially when opioids are involved.

From an integrative medicine approach, the ultimate goal of treatment
is to activate and support the body's natural ability for self-healing, and
to remove any obstacles to this process. For example, when someone
is depressed, they may feel tired, lethargic, and without appetite. An
antidepressant medication may improve their mood, energy level, and
appetite. I believe medication can serve as a bridge to an experiential
reference point for feeling differently. My experience is that the self-healing
techniques of this program may help the patient feel sufficiently better so
that, in time, they may not need the antidepressant.

Oftentimes, when a patient tells me that their pain medication isn't
working, I suspect they had unrealistic expectations of it. Many medicines
used for chronic pain are not intended to make the pain disappear. Rather,
the goal is to reduce the frequency, intensity, or intrusiveness of the pain.
The patients were expecting the pill to make the pain disappear entirely,
and it didn't do that. This may be an issue of inappropriate expectations
for what the medication is supposed to do.

*(List your medications, as well as whether the medications have met your
expectations for relief and improvement)*

Tell me about your family. Are you married/single/divorced? How are your important family relationships going? Do you have friendships? Social supports? How do the people closest to you respond when you are in pain? Are they sympathetic and doting, or more distant and uninterested?

A vast body of research informs us that having the optimal level of social support and interaction is vitally important for healing from chronic pain. The actual amount of sufficient interaction varies from person to person. Optimal interaction for an extrovert may mean meeting with groups of three or four friends at least two or three times per week. But an introvert may be satisfied meeting one close friend once a week. That's because extroverts get energized by spending time with others, while introverts get energized by having time alone. What matters is the quality of these social connections, and how they fit your individual needs—not the number of people you spend time with.

Dr. Stephen Porges's Polyvagal Theory is an important contribution to the literature on the physiology of responses to trauma. The continuum of responses ranges from the fight/flight response to the freeze/faint response. Importantly, he notes that the most adaptive level of response is the social engagement system. When we can respond to and interact with others, it helps us to cope more effectively with difficult situations—such as chronic pain. The social engagement response is more adaptive than lapsing into the fight/flight or freeze/withdrawal responses.

Support from a spouse, family member, or close friend may be crucially important for the healing process. This is especially true when the support person encourages the sufferer to engage in self-care.

It is important to evaluate how the people closest to you respond when you are in pain. Are they more or less likely to respond, compared to when you are feeling well? When a close support treats a chronic pain sufferer in the "sick role," they have a much higher likelihood of increased pain and prolonged suffering. For example, I once saw a patient at a pain clinic who had chronic neck and shoulder pain. Her husband was with her at the appointment. Every time she needed to reach for her water glass or a tissue, her husband would leap out of his chair to get it for her. When I asked him why he did this, he responded, "To save her from pain and suffering." Of course he was trying to be helpful, but he was inadvertently conveying the message to his wife that she was fragile and needed to avoid any unnecessary movement. This is an example of enabling behavior that causes difficulty. Modifying these interpersonal patterns can help the healing process.

(List your most important social and family supports. How do they respond when you are in pain?)

_____

_____

_____

_____

_____

_____

_____

_____

_____

_____

_____

Are you in a chronic pain support group? Do you find it helpful?

Support is important in coping with pain, but the type of support makes a big difference. Well-run support groups encourage participants to actively take care of themselves to get better. This empowers them. However, support groups that cultivate a victim mentality may disempower participants. Some research indicates that such groups may unwittingly increase the pain and suffering of their members. Try to avoid groups that foster a mindset of, "It's us against the world, because nobody else understands us."

(Are you in a chronic pain support group? Please describe whether you find it helpful or not and why.)

_____

_____

_____

_____

_____

_____

_____

_____

_____

Tell me about your work life. What is your job? [If not employed, how do you spend your day? And how are you financially supporting yourself?] How long have you been at this job? Do you like your work? Do you find that the physical demands of your work affect your symptoms? What about the mental/emotional demands?

We spend half of our waking hours at our job, so it is an important setting for people with chronic pain. A lot depends on whether you like your job and find it meaningful. If work is unsatisfying and frustrating, the chronic pain sufferer may find that the pain increases readily during the workday. A job where you feel comfortable will be less of an obstacle to your rehabilitation.

It becomes a rather complex issue if you were injured on the job and receive workers' compensation. On one hand, if someone is injured on the job, they deserve support and compensation. On the other hand, the medical literature informs us that injured workers are not always committed to healing, because once they feel better, they lose their compensation.

Another issue has to do with the physical/mental/emotional demands of the job. Is there physical wear and tear from the actual biomechanical demands of the work? Do the emotional pressures of the job accumulate and make you feel worse? Do the pressures and responsibilities of the job extend beyond your work hours?

(Are you working? If so, what is your job? Do you like it? How do the demands of work affect your pain?)

How do others at work respond to you when you have symptoms?

Just as family and friends play a role in your healing process, so do coworkers. How the people at work respond to you when you are in pain can be important. Do they dote on you and show concern? Or do they ignore you and show indifference to your pain?

_____

_____

_____

_____

_____

_____

_____

_____

_____

_____

_____

_____

_____

What is your level of tension/distress/anxiety/despair *about* your pain right now, 0–10?

Are you clear on the difference between pain and suffering? Suffering is a reaction to pain. It is not easy to distinguish them at first. For example, a patient with low back pain said to me, "The shooting pain in my low back is at a 10 out of 10—I'm overtaken by anxiety and despair. They happen immediately, at the same moment." Only later in treatment was he able to say, "Although the back pain is at a 6 out of 10, my anxiety and despair about it are at a 2 out of 10. It doesn't feel as overwhelming and domineering right now."

A good illustration involved an eighty-six-year-old patient. Her exaggerated curvature of the spine (kyphosis) was so severe that she walked with her head and torso tilted forward almost at a ninety-degree angle. At the beginning of treatment, she rated her pain intensity at 8.5 out of 10, and her despair and hopelessness about her pain was a 10 out of 10. At the end of treatment, the pain intensity dropped to a 5 out of 10. But her despair and hopelessness about the pain went way down, to 2 out of 10. Clearly, she made the distinction between the pain itself and how much it was invading her life.

(What is the level of distress in response to your pain right now? Can you identify what difficult emotions you are experiencing in response to your pain? Or do the pain and suffering still feel like one inseparable overwhelm?)

How has your life changed as a result of the pain? What activities do you have to reduce or avoid because of pain?

Chronic pain is life changing. All too often, nobody asks the patient how their life has changed because of the pain. How has the pain altered their self-identity? How much anger/shame/grief is attached to their pain at this point?

An example of the life-changing thrust of chronic pain is the story of my patient Corrine Before her migraines, Connie used to feel happy and carefree. She was creative, inspired, and full of energy. But then came the chronic headache pain. It hung around her like an albatross, weighing her down with a burden of guilt. Pain had changed her life so much that she felt as if she was letting down family and coworkers—falling short both at work and at home. Sometimes she wondered whether her life was worth living.

Other patients have felt broken, as if to say, "My body is damaged goods and doesn't work properly. I don't see anyone else suffering all the time like me."

Still others feel shameful about their symptoms.

A retired postal worker in his mid-fifties with chronic leg and foot pain told me, "My father complained about his back pain as far back as I can remember. He never held down a job because of it, and he never had time for me. I always vowed that I would be different from him. When I feel my pain surge, I feel ashamed because it makes me afraid that I'm becoming like my father."

In order to restore your life, you must first understand how chronic pain has taken it away.

(How has your life changed as a result of the pain?)

What is your daily schedule from time of waking to time of going to sleep? Do you take any breaks during the day? [Meals and otherwise]

Over the years, people build up habits for how they spend their time. It becomes like a schedule for the workweek and weekends. Many hard-working people have learned to keep that schedule in mind regardless of how bad they feel. They disconnect their head from their body and just keep pushing themselves through their work and tasks every day. This becomes problematic when you suffer from chronic pain.

One of the most difficult changes for some chronic pain sufferers to accept is that their pain has finally required them to change how they pace themselves. For some people, this question may be the first time they have ever considered how they pace themselves through the day.

Despite his neck and shoulder pain, my patient Jeff stuck to his daily routine: "I get up at six o'clock, grab a cup of coffee to go on my way to the office. At the office by seven, spend much of my day in a cubicle staring at a computer screen. I may grab a donut in the break room, but otherwise I'm working straight though lunch except for coffee—there's too much in my inbox. I don't take any breaks because I'm trying to get ahead on tasks, and besides, my supervisor is keeping track of when I'm working and when I'm on a break. I leave the office by around six thirty or seven. Getting home, I'll usually have one or two glasses of wine to unwind. Typically I'll bring in fast food for dinner, because who has time to cook? Then I'll unwind in front of the boob tube for a few hours. I'll go to bed around midnight, but first I have another glass of wine just to help me relax enough to get sleepy. And by the way—don't ask me to take more breaks, because I'll be under so much more pressure at work that I'll feel much worse!"

Like many of my chronic pain patients, Jeff's workday pace and lack of self-care contribute greatly to his ongoing pain. It's very hard to change those patterns when someone who is facing so many demands is simply trying their best to get through the day.

(List what hours you work during the day, and the time/length of any breaks you take.)

How is your sleep? Any problems with initial/middle/terminal insomnia? Apnea? Do you awaken because of the pain, or does the awakening seem separate from pain? Is your sleep non-rejuvenative?

Sleep problems are so common in chronic pain that it is rare when a pain sufferer does *not* have trouble sleeping. This problem is so important that I devote an entire section to it later in this book (see "Awareness of Your Sleep," from the "Awareness" chapter).

How often do you drink alcohol? What is your typical use, and what is the most you might consume in a day? Any problems or treatment for alcohol abuse or dependency? Any use of marijuana [Medical or recreational]? What happens to your symptoms when you use alcohol or marijuana?

For many people, it is common to have a glass of wine or a beer or two on a weekend night, often with friends, but some chronic pain sufferers turn to alcohol for pain relief. This is a false promise, however, as alcohol causes far more problems for the pain sufferer than it solves. It is a diuretic, meaning that it depletes water from the body. Dehydration can make chronic pain feel worse. Alcohol often interacts negatively with many common pain medications, causing fatigue, brain fog, and other problems. It encourages disconnection from bodily sensations, which can lead you to lose touch with somatic cues that signal when you need rest, stretching, or other self-care. Use of beer, wine, or hard liquor to help you sleep actually disturbs your sleep cycle and makes sleep more difficult. And, of course, use of alcohol to cope with pain can lead to alcohol dependence.

In recent months, there has been an explosion of media attention about the use of marijuana and cannabidiol (CBD) for treating everything under the sun, including chronic pain. CBD is the second most prevalent active ingredient in marijuana. Much research is currently being done to investigate the effectiveness of CBD for treating chronic pain. The current evidence suggests that there may be clinical benefit, but we are still early in our understanding of how it works, what drug interactions exist, and which types of pain respond best to CBD. Whether using CBD, medical marijuana, or recreational marijuana, it is important to discuss the frequency and circumstances of your use of it. Many of the same concerns for using alcohol also exist when using marijuana. From a scientific standpoint, we do not yet know conclusively what its impact is. It's important to discuss CBD usage with your health provider.

(How often do you use alcohol, marijuana or CBD?)

Have you ever suffered from psychological problems such as depression, anxiety, trauma, phobias, or marital or family problems? Have you ever received psychological treatment or psychotherapy for this? Medication?

We have already discussed how chronic pain patients often feel defensive about the implication that their symptoms are psychosomatic. This defensiveness is understandable, even after assuring you that your chronic pain is real and not "just in your head."

Although this can be a touchy issue, it is important to inquire about any psychological problems. That's because research tells us that depression, anxiety, or previous traumatic events can physically worsen your pain. Do a quick gut check: How do you feel about this topic? Open? Defensive? Confused? It needs to be discussed because, if you suffer from some of these issues, it will affect your pain treatment. Besides, it is quite common to feel depressed, anxious, or traumatized when struggling with chronic pain.

It's also important to discuss any medications you may be taking to treat depression or anxiety. Many of these medications are also prescribed for treating chronic pain. Do you feel these medications are helping you? How are the side effects? There is a vicious cycle at work here. Depression makes pain feel more intense, and of course, the pain itself can be depressing.

Have you ever had thoughts of not wanting to live anymore?

This is a very sensitive topic, one that people do not want to discuss. Yet it is very important that we do discuss it. I have met so many people with chronic pain whose lives have been turned upside-down with suffering, agony, and loss. If you have had these thoughts, know that you are not alone. Studies have shown that up to 30 percent of chronic pain patients have had at least fleeting thoughts of suicide. This reflects the profound level of suffering associated with chronic pain. We can do much together to address this issue, and it starts with being able to talk about it. *(NOTE: If you are currently experiencing suicidal thoughts, please let somebody know **now**, such as your spouse and/or your primary care provider.)*

What do you imagine your life would be like if your pain never went away? Conversely, what do you imagine your life would be like if the pain disappeared tomorrow? What would be different in your home life, work life, relationships, and sense of self, and what you would do differently in your day?

In my more than thirty years of treating chronic pain, I have seen a common pattern where patients over time tend to "hunker down" with their burden of pain. You learn to grit your teeth and bear it over the long haul. You tend to numb yourself to the day's demands, just trying to make it through. You don't even consider the worst-case scenario of what life might be like if this awful pain never goes away. Nevertheless, your body carries the emotional reverberation of these fears. You also don't allow yourself to indulge in the luxury of imagining how much easier life would be without the burden of pain. You don't allow yourself to picture what wishes and dreams you would be following if you only felt well enough to do so. Would you start riding your bike every day? Would you go out dancing with your husband? Would you enjoy the return of sexual desire with your partner if you were not burdened with chronic low back pain? Would you take more vacations to see your grandchildren? What are the things that you want and need to do for yourself that you don't even let yourself think about because of the constant albatross of pain?

It is important to shine a spotlight upon these hopes and wishes and fears and aspirations. They provide clues to how the burden of chronic pain has uniquely affected you. They point to what changes we need to pursue to help you regain your life.

(What do you imagine your life would be like if your pain never went away?)

[What do you imagine your life would be like if your pain disappeared tomorrow?]

I suggest that you bring this completed pain assessment to the health providers that are treating your chronic pain. Your answers will help you and your clinicians to treat your pain more effectively.

This pain assessment is now completed. As we said, the assessment is the beginning of treatment. Hopefully these questions have stimulated your thinking in ways that might be new and different. These questions give clues about some of the variables that will be important to pursue in the ABC treatment program that lies ahead.

CHAPTER 11

Your Healing Map: What Does the Healing Process Look Like?

"HOW LONG IS THIS GOING TO TAKE?"

As you now embark on the process of healing, I have found that it is indispensable to have a roadmap for how healing will progress. There are ups and downs to be sure, but the ultimate trajectory should be heading in a positive direction. What I have seen in many years of clinical practice is that most chronic pain patients don't know what to expect as they work on rehabilitation. Some of the questions I often hear are, "How long is this going to take?" "I should be much better by now and I'm not," or "How come I work on all these exercises and I still feel pain?"

Once you have gone through the process of learning about your chronic pain, you have found a team of trusted professionals, you trust your diagnosis and have proceeded from the diagnostic phase to the rehabilitation phase—now what?

One of the purposes of this section is to provide you with appropriate expectations for the healing process. Why? Because the expectations you have about healing will affect all aspects of your rehabilitation.

Surprisingly, even though almost 20 percent of the US population suffers at some point with chronic pain, there is little or no information out there about how the healing process progresses over time when someone has chronic pain. A Google search today on that topic reveals all kinds of suggestions for various treatments (physical therapy, medications, acupuncture), but nothing about what to expect on the road to healing.

So, let's discuss it now.

PAIN DISTORTS TIME

Of course, whenever we are in pain, it's natural to want it to *go away—NOW!* Hypnosis research informs us that we perceive time as passing more slowly when we are in pain. This phenomenon—known as time distortion—makes the pain sufferer inherently impatient for relief. At the same time, it is important to understand that we can be patient and that the progress will still move forward.

THE POWER OF YOUR EXPECTATIONS

We already know that your expectations affect your experience. This relates to the well–researched area of placebos. Any FDA–approved medication must successfully be shown effective in *placebo-controlled* research (where the effects of a drug are compared to the effects of a placebo and shown to be superior). Why is this necessary? Because we know that one's expectation of help from a drug is such a powerful influencer that it accounts from anywhere from *33 to 40 percent of a drug's efficacy!* One's positive—or negative—expectation of a drug or other treatment will affect how much or little benefit they receive, regardless of the biological impact.

It turns out that expectation also changes how your brain and spinal cord perceive pain.

One aspect of how pain is processed and perceived is called *descending analgesia* (DA). DA means that nerve pathways descending from the brain down into the spinal cord sometimes inhibit the intensity of pain signals that are registered and felt. For example, one of the ways that analgesic pain medications work is by triggering DA. Several years ago, an article was published in the *Journal of Pain* entitled "Descending Analgesia—When the Spine Echoes what the Brain Expects." It revealed that, when someone expects that a treatment or activity will lead to pain relief, areas of the brainstem send signals downward to the spinal cord, producing decreased pain. Conversely, when someone expects that a treatment or activity will lead to pain worsening, these protective descending signals from the brain are limited, leading to increased feeling of pain.

So, we want to take advantage of having good, solid, helpful expectations for how healing will progress.

When I played competitive tennis, my coach used to push me to improve my forehand and backhand strokes for maximum power and efficiency. When I hit the ball right in the "sweet spot" in the center of the racquet, it made this wonderful "thwack" sound that meant I was hitting it with speed and power. Your rehabilitation will consist of focusing on several different areas of skills. Stretching and muscle strengthening. Somatic awareness. Emotional awareness. Pacing skills. Calming and quieting skills. Physical conditioning. Your goal here as well is to find your "sweet spot"—in other words, learning to gauge how much or little to push yourself. If you don't exercise enough, you won't make enough forward progress. But if you exercise too much or too hard, you may injure yourself and set back the healing process. With time and practice, working with your healing team, you will find your "sweet spot" for pacing your rehabilitation.

TWO STEPS FORWARD, ONE STEP BACK

I have found that the way we are hardwired to rehabilitate from chronic pain is a process of "two steps forward, one step back." It's as if we make some progress, and then sometimes we slip back a little, almost as if our body and mind take a step back for a moment to absorb and incorporate the change we just made. Here in Minnesota, where we have very snowy winters and our cars get stuck, my patients understand the adage, "Sometimes you have to put the car in reverse for a few seconds in order to shift forward and get out of the rut!"

Remember that in chronic pain, the ultimate goal may not be the complete disappearance of all pain. When it comes to healing from chronic pain, the community standard for improvement is a reduction in the frequency, intensity, and intrusiveness of your pain. This means that, although you may have (for example) some remnants of low back pain over time, you'll find that you have pain episodes less often, they hurt less, and they interfere less and less with your returning to normal activities that you enjoy.

Once you are aware of how the healing process progresses with chronic pain, this will reduce your feelings of frustration, anger, despair, and hopelessness. You will likely breathe a sigh of relief and find yourself being a little more patient with the process. And as you feel more patient, your autonomic nervous system will become less agitated and dysregulated in response to feeling pain sensations as well, further reducing your pain along the healing path.

DEEP HEALING TAKES TIME

Healing from a chronic illness (such as chronic pain) takes longer than healing from acute illness. This makes sense. As humans, we develop a relationship with anything that has been with us over time. When you have experienced low back pain for at least three to six months, your relationship to it can't help but change. You start to walk differently, perhaps tightening and bracing your hips, buttocks, pelvic floor, and leg muscles to instinctively guard the painful areas. Your nervous system becomes sensitized by then, so that previously neutral sensations may now feel painful. Changing these patterns takes more time compared to someone who injured their back two weeks ago.

So, the healing process takes time, and there are inevitably setbacks. Even when you move ahead with a reasonable, balanced program of rehabilitation, you will likely experience an occasional flare episode. Most of my patients find that dealing with a flare episode is one of the most difficult parts of the healing process. While upsetting, flares are normal and common, and there are proven strategies to help you get through them successfully. (See Chapter 25: "Eight Steps for Handling a Pain Flare.")

THE GOAL OF ALL TREATMENTS

Ultimately, all pain treatments you participate in are working gradually to help you access your own inherent internal self-healing resources. Every treatment you undergo, every self-care activity you practice, should be directed toward this goal. For example, you may be taking medication to reduce pain, ease anxiety, calm down an agitated nervous system, or help you sleep better. The appropriate expectation for taking an analgesic pain medication may *not* be to make the pain disappear. Rather, the appropriate expectation for the drug is that it will reduce the intensity of the pain enough for you to catch your breath. To help you "untie your hands from behind your back" so that you can more effectively utilize your own skills and tools for dealing with the pain (such as breathing techniques, grounding, journal writing, gentle exercise, and so on).

A patient of mine healing from chronic head and neck pain recently said to me: "As a senior vice president of a large company and a serious marathon runner, I've been accustomed to pushing myself at 110 percent and expecting quick results. Get the job done, and fast. When I work on something hard and the problem isn't completely solved, I feel like I've become weak and lazy. I feel ashamed. I feel that I have failed."

Without milestones along the way, the task can feel overwhelming. To heal from a chronic condition over time, you must be able to feel that you are making progress along the way. How you view your pain and your expectations are important here as well, because this will affect whether you feel you are progressing or not.

Denise, a thirty-three-year-old patient suffering from fibromyalgia, struggled with pain in her neck, shoulders, arms, thighs, and shins. On this particular day in my office, she rated the intensity of her aching pain at a 6 out of 10. We then did a brief self-hypnosis for calming and pain relief. When we finished, she said, "It didn't help, and I'm not improving!" I asked her to rate the pain intensity after the hypnosis, and she said, "3 out of 10." Surprised, I commented, "So that means that your pain intensity reduced to about one-half of where it was before you did the hypnosis." She replied, "Yes—but I don't consider the pain improved unless it's *gone*."

For Denise, it was an all-or-nothing proposition. Either her pain has entirely disappeared, or else it's as if nothing has changed at all.

While it may be understandable that someone who has been suffering from pain for years would want it completely gone so badly, viewing the healing process in this all-or-nothing way is unrealistic, and certainly counterproductive.

Since chronic pain has taken at least three to six months to develop, I think it's reasonable to think that it will take around that same length of time to rehabilitate well. You will certainly experience improvements within the first month, but it will likely take three to six months for more prolonged, sustainable progress. Of course, the details of your particular chronic pain symptoms will affect how long rehabilitation takes.

Instead, the golden path to healing from chronic pain is to notice and acknowledge small, incremental improvements along the way. If you do a breathing technique and the ache in your legs drops from a 4 out of 10 to a 3 out of 10, that's a change! If you are having trouble sleeping and you can stay asleep twenty minutes longer than you did last night, that's an improvement! If you are on a walking program to heal from chronic fatigue syndrome and you were able to walk for three blocks instead of two, celebrate it!

HEALING FROM CHRONIC PAIN:
AN ATHLETIC ENDEAVOR

Because of the physical, mental, and emotional demands of rehabilitation, I have found it to be very similar to getting in training for an athletic event. When a long–distance runner is on a track team, training for the season's events, he knows that he doesn't just run and do exercises for a week or two and then compete. Instead, he comes to practice every day. The aim is to get stronger and better over time, a little bit more every week. If he loses a competition or gets injured, his coach and his team remind him that "staying on track" with slow and steady progress is the path to success. He does his running drills. He also works with his coach. He works on improving his form, his technique, his endurance. His coach also works with him on strength training. He reminds him about proper nutrition and getting enough quality rest.

Think of me, and your healing team, as your "coaching staff." Stick with the ABC plan, and with time and practice you will reach your healing goals!

THE ABC METHOD
Awareness, Balancing, and Cultivating

SECTION III

Awareness

Introduction
to Awareness

Awareness is the cornerstone of the ABC method. You can't change anything if you don't first see it, sense it, or feel it. The ability to pay attention to your sensations and emotions is a foundational skill for healing from chronic pain. And yet, it can be a challenging skill to acquire. Learning to focus your awareness is the beginning of the process of creating healing changes in your body. Awareness sounds easy. Like the pain patient who said to me "Oh, I'm aware of my pain all right—I'm aware of it all the time, day and night, more aware than I *want* to be."

Joanne, a patient of mine with chronic abdominal pain, walked into my office for an appointment. She announced that she was feeling fairly relaxed that day. I noticed immediately that her forehead was tightened, jaw clenched, and shoulders hunched up toward her ears. When I pointed out the possibility that she might be experiencing tension outside her awareness, she replied, "But, Dr. Weisberg—I'm not tense!"

Joanne wasn't lying to me, either. To the best of her knowledge and awareness, she wasn't sensing any tension. The tension was there, but she was oblivious to it. Had she noticed, she could have taken advantage of that sensory awareness as a prompt to take some action to feel better, such as a brief stretch or a breathing technique.

AWARENESS CAN BE ELUSIVE

Establishing awareness as a skill can feel elusive, and at times tricky. For example, have you ever sat in a room for a long time, but not noticed the sound of the overhead ventilation system until someone pointed it out? The noise had been in the background the whole time.

A central tenet of integrative medicine is that the body is not stupid! Symptoms are *intelligent* signals trying to get our attention. We just need to learn how to listen to them. There is a physiological basis to understanding symptoms and sensations as messages. It has to do with the ways that your sensations, emotions, thoughts, and moods affect your pain.

AWARENESS: LIKE LEARNING TO PLAY A NEW SPORT

If you have ever learned a new athletic skill, like a tennis forehand, a golf swing, or even a new dance step, you may have noticed mild soreness the next day. Your coach guided you to make new movements and use muscles that you weren't used to using. Developing awareness is no different. The skills needed to exercise this kind of awareness may feel new, novel, like you've never used them before. Learning to develop awareness is similar to the skills exercised by a quarterback, a baseball pitcher, or a point guard on a basketball team. The pitcher learns to notice slight variations in the stance of the batter at the plate before throwing a curve ball. The golfer attends to subtleties in the wind velocity and direction before her shot.

So what does the language of your body sound like? What does it feel like? What are its rhythms, cadences, intensity, and volume? Noticing them requires slowing down and then intentionally focusing your attention. You may find that your mind is restless, seemingly too busy all day for even fifteen seconds of slow breathing. Perhaps silence and awareness are a bit too uncomfortable. Keeping your brain busy and distracted is how you've learned to cope—by remaining completely oblivious to inner messages. This is something you can learn to change.

AWARENESS AND THE PROBLEM
OF NORMAL DISSOCIATION

Dissociation is the act of disconnecting things. It is the opposite of association, which brings things together. Your mind *dis-associates* from things it finds uncomfortable. It does this by blocking awareness of unpleasant sensations or feelings. Dissociation is the opposite of awareness. It is the blocking of awareness, a power to ignore things. It is a very common feature of the mind, and it often plays a negative role in cases of chronic pain.

Dissociation ranges across a continuum from a useful coping mechanism to a severe disorder. An extreme case of dissociation is what used to be called multiple personality disorder. The most famous case of this disorder is the story of Sybil, a pseudonym for a patient who was said to have sixteen distinct personalities. Her therapist concluded that all these different personalities were a result of severe child sex abuse. The various personalities gave Sybil a way to disconnect from this trauma. Her story became a bestselling book in the 1970s and spawned two made-for-TV-movies.

Another famous story of dissociation comes from a novel by Robert Louis Stevenson, *The Strange Case of Dr. Jekyll and Mr. Hyde*. Numerous movies and parodies have been based on this nineteenth-century tale of a man who split into two distinct personalities. The good Dr. Jekyll would transform into the evil Mr. Hyde, but neither personality was aware of the other.

Another popular type of dissociation can be found in the world of sports. We read all the time about athletes who get injured during a game but play on anyway. You know, the star quarterback is sacked and fractures his collarbone in the third quarter. But he gets up and goes on to win the game. The intense pain doesn't surface until the final whistle blows. A similar case is the soldier who is wounded in combat but doesn't feel the searing pain until hours later, when he has made it to safety. It's like the title of Jesse Ventura's autobiography, *I Ain't Got Time to Bleed*.

In the midst of important action, these figures disassociate themselves from feeling pain.

Less heroic forms of dissociation are a normal part of daily life. Daydreaming while you are driving is a common way to disconnect from the boredom of a routine activity. More broadly, we all dissociate as a way to cope with painful and uncomfortable experiences virtually every day. We may ignore a rude remark from a coworker just to avoid the irritation. You may put off thinking about a decision with your spouse for fear it will spiral into an argument.

Another rationale for dissociation is to disconnect with physical discomfort. We are bombarded daily with TV commercials that remind us of this. "Don't let back pain interfere with your day—take Advil and get on with life." We also self-medicate. A beer or a glass of wine after work serves for many people as a way to disconnect from the fatigue and physical tension of the day.

And of course, let's not forget one of the most common forms of distraction: our cell phones. It's increasingly common that when you encounter a group of people, the majority of them are looking at their phones. They are constantly attentive to their notifications, checking the latest texts and email, and finding out what's new on Instagram, Tik Tok, Twitter, and Facebook. We see so many patients at our pain clinic suffering from the physical effects of this habit that we came up with a new diagnosis: "Turtle-ing!" The characteristic stance while checking your phone is to jut your head forward and down, with shoulders rolled and hunched forward, just like a turtle. This odd posture has become an increasingly common cause of head and neck pain.

DISSOCIATION AND CHRONIC PAIN

It is normal to disconnect from the experience of chronic pain. As many patients have told me over the years, "You can't blame me for abandoning my body when it has been ravaged by pain!"

Some types of disconnection can be harmless, but dissociation can be a real problem when treating chronic pain. It is so common because we have a natural tendency to avoid pain. We consider it a threat. The injured football player only has to make it until the end of the game, but people with chronic pain have to cope with it all day long, every day. They feel a need to disconnect from a constant pain that is frustrating and exhausting.

One dissociative strategy is to avoid using the painful part of the body. Someone with chronic pain in the left arm may actually stop using the entire left side of their body. This may seem like overkill, but once again it is a natural tendency to brace the entire area just to protect the painful spot. We instinctively guard an injured back by finding a safe position and trying not to move from it. Guarding sends the message: "Don't move a muscle until that low back is better!" We guard in order to prevent our muscles from moving and aggravating the injury. It is as if the brain preempts any risky movements by triggering pain and tension before the movement actually takes place. If any movement occurs in the guarded area, you get anxious. All of this aggravates the pain sensation itself. This cycle of guarding/dissociation/avoidance/anxiety/pain is all too common in chronic pain. Despite the good intentions, this strategy backfires—because it prolongs the suffering.

When dissociating from pain becomes a habit, patients have difficulty being aware of the feelings in their body in general. By blocking somatic sensations, they miss all the nuances, as well as any changes in sensation. This is one reason why so many chronic pain patients have difficulty learning relaxation techniques. Since they have trouble noticing changes before and after doing these techniques, they are oblivious to any improvements. This convinces them that the exercises are useless.

Another reason that dissociation and guarding is a problem is because our body is designed to move. Normal movement facilitates multiple self-healing mechanisms in our body. Awareness of bodily sensations can help us to stay healthy by reminding us to move. For example, noticing stiffness at the base of the neck provides a cue for us to stop and stretch the tight areas. This feels good, and prevents the subsequent development of a muscle tension headache.

TAKING SIDES

George had an intense burning pain in his right arm and hand that had persisted for over seven years. Although George was right-handed, he started performing all simple actions with his left hand. Whether he was shaking hands, opening a door, turning on a light, or even tossing a ball— he always did it left-handed. One time I watched George walk down a hallway. His left arm would swing back and forth normally, but his right arm just hung there, practically motionless. I'm sure he began just by disconnecting from the painful sensations in his arm, but he progressively disowned the entire right side of his torso!

Part of George's healing process involved learning to reclaim the right side of his body from the waist up. He needed to become less fearful and more accepting of that side of his body. Slowly and gradually, George began to reconnect with the feelings in his right arm, starting with becoming aware of mild, neutral sensations.

SENSORY AWARENESS:
POSITIVE NEUROPLASTICITY

As we discussed earlier, neuroplasticity can be either a friend or foe in the process of healing from chronic pain. Dissociation that hinders healing is a form of negative neuroplasticity.

To correct this habit, George needed to develop the positive habit of sensory awareness and somatic monitoring. In other words, developing the ability to notice the sensations of his body, and then noticing changes in those sensations. These essential skills promote the healing process and enable neuroplasticity to work for George instead of against him. He could make no progress in his rehabilitation until he could observe those milder sensations—*before* they intensified to the point of pain.

Decreasing dissociation is one reason why sensory awareness is an important part of my ABC method for treating chronic pain. You need to become more comfortable with paying attention to all kinds of sensory experience in the body, especially the dissociated or disowned parts.

How do you do this? One example of developing this skill is learning to tell the difference between what a tight muscle feels like versus a loose muscle. Or what it feels like when your shoulders are clenched up toward your ears versus when they are back down in a relaxed position. Ultimately, it means learning to recognize the state of your autonomic nervous system. Notice whether your nervous system is revving up or winding down. Compare that to when you feel centered.

The development of such awareness doesn't happen instantly. Like many skills you'll learn in the ABC method, it will take time and practice to make it second nature. Paradoxically, when you start practicing awareness, you may feel a little worse at first. That's because you will start feeling the underlying pain and discomfort that you were successfully avoiding for months or years. Rest assured that this expanded awareness will soon lead to a decrease in your pain.

CHAPTER 12

Awareness of Your Sensations, Emotions, and Thoughts

When it comes to understanding how we experience chronic pain, we need to turn our attention to the way that our brain reflects pain in our body.

Our brain not only perceives—it also predicts.

Until recently, our thinking has been that the brain is an organ that accurately reflects and reacts to stimuli from the outside world. For example, if a glass pitcher falls from a table near you, your brain allows you to hear, see, and feel the impact. However, if you are watching a movie scene where a glass pitcher falls from a table but the sound is off, your brain can still generate a version of these sensations. Therefore, you may be startled at the scene of a glass pitcher falling off a table even though you don't hear it or feel the vibration of the shattering glass hitting the ground.

What does this mean? It reflects that our brain helps us perceive the world around us by combining sensory information in the moment with *memories* of similar experiences from the past and anticipation of how the pain will be in the future. In other words, our brain not only perceives—it also predicts. This is why, for example, many people flinch when they are about to receive a shot at the doctor's office. They haven't even had the needle puncture their skin, but their brain is already predicting pain, based on earlier memories of needles.

Similarly, someone suffering for years from chronic low back pain who experiences a twinge of discomfort may feel more than strictly the result of a tight muscle and irritated sciatic nerves. The pain experience is also colored by a brain which both predicts how severe the pain will be and remembers past memories of similar painful experiences. The sum total is a combination of past pain and predicted future pain, as well as the effect of strained muscles and nerves in the present moment.

It is indeed amazing how our brain remembers the past and predicts the future, to help us effectively perceive the world. But it causes a major problem for chronic pain sufferers. Feeling the ache of chronic neck pain, the stab of chronic migraine pain, or the pulsing twist of low back pain is bad enough. But when your brain adds to this by remembering past incidents of overwhelming pain and projecting expectation of future suffering, the net result can be overwhelming. This is where state–dependent memory (refer to chapter "The Science of Chronic Pain," p. 27) can wreak havoc on the chronic pain sufferer. The more the pain is amplified by past memories and future expectations of pain, the worse the cycles of chronic suffering become.

There is a way to break these vicious cycles of pain and suffering. The goal is to curb your brain's tendency to respond to pain with bad memories and predictions of distress. This requires training your brain to bring its attention to the sensations and thoughts of the moment.

SENSORY AWARENESS, EMOTIONAL AWARENESS, AND THOUGHT (COGNITIVE) AWARENESS OF CHRONIC PAIN

Chronic pain affects us powerfully and simultaneously on the levels of sensation, emotion, and thought. To make sense of the experience of chronic pain and to establish tools for coping, we need to first break this phenomenon down into its component parts. We will first look at each one of these dimensions separately, to get to know and observe them more effectively. Finally, I will show you how to bring awareness to the sensations, emotions, and thoughts that comprise your experience of chronic pain.

SENSATION

Sensation refers to the physical feeling in your body. When you are in pain, some of those sensations may include aching, tingling, burning, stabbing, tight, electric, buzzing, numb, muffled, fuzzy, raw. It's important to remember that you may perceive multiple sensations simultaneously.

Some people feel flooded with sensations throughout the day and night. Others may actually have difficulty identifying a sensation in their body. The goal is to be able to notice various sensations as they occur in your body. Not just "thinking about" the sensation (as in, "I know I feel this aching pain all the time"), but paying attention to it right now, in real time.

For all the following brief exercises, have either a pen and paper or a laptop computer close by so you can record what you start to notice.

Brief Exercise for Somatic Awareness

Sit in a comfortable chair. Notice a neutral sensation somewhere in your body. It might be the feeling of your forearm and hand resting on your leg. It might be the feeling of some part of the chair resting against your back or seat. Or it might be a mild tingling or warmth in your foot or your thigh. Just observe the sensation, describe how strong the sensation is (from 1 being extremely mild to 10 being extremely intense). Make a brief notation marking this.

EMOTION

Examples of emotions include happy, sad, angry, bored, irritated, betrayed, ashamed, excited, tender. These can be triggered by something external in the present (such as a stressful day at work) or by something internal (such as an unpleasant memory or ongoing patterns of perceiving yourself negatively).

Remember that the only place that we can perceive emotion is in the body. Fear may manifest as tingling in the stomach. Excitement reveals itself as a quickened heart rate. Anger presents with your jaw stiffening, or a surge of energy up your spine. Sadness may appear as a heaviness in the chest.

Brief Exercise for Emotional Awareness

Sit down with a piece of paper and pen. Take a few slow deep breaths. Ask yourself, "What am I feeling emotionally right now?" Allow a few minutes if necessary for the awareness of the feeling(s) to emerge. Some examples may include, "I feel···tired, weary, tense, happy, hopeful, anxious, etc." Write this feeling down, without any need to explain "why" you feel the particular emotion.

As a variation on the above exercise, identify the emotion connected to your chronic pain. Start by identifying the area of pain in your body (for example, a moderate feeling of aching in your legs). Then, ask yourself, "What emotion do I feel in response to this leg pain being here right now?" Allow time for the awareness of the feelings to emerge. Again, write the feeling down, without any need to explain "why" you feel it.

THOUGHT

A thought is a mental experience, a mental image, a memory, or a string of words. Our ideas, opinions, and beliefs about ourselves. Thoughts are racing through our minds all the time, often hiding in the background under our conscious awareness. They are, however, coloring our perceptions of ourselves as well as of our pain.

What makes these thoughts more problematic is that over time they become more automatic and may often continue below our conscious awareness. In other words, "under the radar." The goal, with practice, is two-fold. First, to bring conscious awareness to the thoughts that have been recurring under the radar, so that you can be aware of what has been affecting you. Second, being aware of these thoughts opens the opportunity to provide a rational alternative. For example, once you are aware that you have concluded that a worse headache means there is no hope, you can respond with the statement that says, "Even though my headache is worse today, I have often felt the pain improve the next day, and it can improve again."

Brief Exercise for Thought Awareness

Sit in a comfortable chair. Take a few deep breaths. Start to listen in to the ongoing noise of your thoughts. As soon as you begin to notice some of the thoughts, stop for a moment and jot them down on laptop or paper.

Examples of thoughts you notice about your pain may include:

- "This exercise is silly—why do I even need it?"

- "This is too much effort."

- "I just remembered I need to pick up cheese and bread at the grocery later."

- "What time is my doctor appointment next week?"

- "Am I doing this exercise properly?"

- "I resent the way my boss scolded me in front of the staff last week."

- "This pain is hopeless—It will never get better."

- "The fact that my headache is worse this week is proof that there is no hope."

- "It doesn't matter that my back pain reduced from a 6 to a 4. It isn't better unless it is entirely gone."

- "I hate this neck pain because it means I'm just like my sick father."

- "I am a failure because I haven't been able to get rid of this chronic joint pain."

The goal, with practice, is to be able to develop the ability to sit back and just observe the ongoing noise of your thoughts without judging them as good or bad.

"DEAR DIARY"–A POWERFUL TOOL FOR BUILDING AWARENESS

Writing in a journal can be a powerful tool for improving your ability to access awareness of your sensations, emotions, and thoughts.

It seems so deceptively simple to think that writing thoughts and feelings in a journal could provide much of any benefit. And yet we now know that journal writing can contribute to profound improvements in emotional and physical health. Journal writing has been demonstrated empirically to reduce chronic pain, improve immune function, decrease stress, improve mood, decrease depression and anxiety, and improve problem-solving skills. It can help you to notice important gradual changes in your symptoms. It can help you to notice side effects caused by your pain, medications, or other interventions. It can help you identify patterns in your pain and identify other potential triggers for your pain symptoms. It can help you to better identify what treatments are helping—or not. And it can help you to provide more accurate communication to your healing team about your progress.

Psychologist Dr. James Pennebaker has done well-designed research on journal writing. He has found that writing in a journal regularly can decrease the symptoms of pain from difficult-to-treat conditions such as rheumatoid arthritis.

When I explain the benefits of journal writing to one of my patients, I often use a metaphor of listening to music. Imagine that you are listening to one of your favorite musical artists in your living room on high-quality headphones. You're really getting into the music, immersed in it. Suddenly you feel a tap on your shoulder, and somebody asks you, "Hey—what are you listening to?" Being able to answer that question requires you to apply a few different types of awareness. First, you need to take a moment and step back from the experience that you were immersed in. Then, you need to be able to tune inside to your feelings to even know what the experience is (e.g., feeling "in the groove," "joyful," "like I gotta dance," etc.). Then, you would need to find the words to express in words what that experience is. "I was listening to my favorite U2 album and I felt so happy and energized!"

Part of what makes journal writing so useful is that it requires the writer to develop these same awareness skills. When you are immersed in the experience of chronic pain, feeling sore, tight, annoyed, and exhausted, imagine how useful it could be to be able to take a step back from the experience and observe it with some distance. And then to be able to tune in and perceive the sensations, emotions, and thoughts going on in that challenging moment. And then, to find the words to accurately describe the experience. This is how journal writing develops indispensable skills for awareness, coping, and healing.

The journal writing that I recommend you do combines awareness of your physical sensations with noticing the emotions, thoughts, and perceptions that occur before, during, and after experiencing pain.

To begin, start by filling in a sheet that lists the following categories:

- Date and time; activities you've been involved in since the last entry

- Where in your body you feel the discomfort

- Whether any self-care activity (e.g., stretching, taking a warm shower, etc.) helped

- What thoughts you have in response to the pain, and what emotions you felt in response to the pain

When you measure the discomfort, remember to use the 0–10 scale we discussed before, where 10 is "the worst pain I have ever experienced" and 0 is "no pain at all."

Then, have another section for brief, freestyle comments. This might include something like, "Today I could sense that my back calmed down a little after practicing the 30-to-1 breathing exercise, and what I feel about that is a little hopeful."

Here is a suggestion to supercharge your journal writing. Be sure to include the feeling associated with whatever you're experiencing. So, instead of writing, "My back pain is at a 5 out of 10 today," write, "My back pain is at a 5 out of 10 today, and what I feel about that is frustration and disappointment." We know from multiple studies of journal writing that the benefits are greatly increased when whatever is described is associated with emotional expression. If you find it difficult to identify which emotions are surfacing for you, start with using the acronym "SASHET," which stands for sad, angry, scared, happy, excited, tender. Of course, this is far from an inclusive list of all emotions, but you may find it to be a helpful starting point.

Like any important new skill, journal writing takes practice, and you'll get better at it as you do it more. Many patients who utilize journal writing as a coping strategy for pain tell me that they start to look forward to their journal writing, feeling like they have another tool to exercise helpful control over their healing.

TYING IT ALL TOGETHER

Now that you have brief exercises and journal writing available to become aware of the sensations, emotions, and thoughts associated with your pain, you can start to use these exercises to disrupt your brain's cycles of remembering and predicting. Doing so will take some of the sting out of your pain episodes.

CHAPTER 13

Awareness of Your Stresses

Stress is a normal and inescapable fact of life. And not all stress is bad. In fact, stress is part of what makes life interesting, challenging, stimulating—up to a point. It's only when stress exceeds a certain threshold that it starts to cause wear and tear. The well-known symptoms of that wear and tear include these:

- Low energy

- Headaches

- Widespread aches and pains

- Muscle tension

- Loss of sexual desire and performance

- Frequent colds and infections

- Upset stomach and disrupted digestion

- Depression and anxiety

- Decreased concentration and attention

- Anxious or racing thoughts

- Eating too much or too little

- Withdrawing from others

- Nervous habits such as nail biting or tooth grinding

- Sleeping too little or too much

By now you should understand that the approach of integrated medicine does not make a sharp distinction between so-called physical and psychological factors. Physical events change our psychological responses, and psychological events lead to physiological changes at the cellular level. Keep in mind that stress is both physical *and* psychological.

In my previous book, *Trust Your Gut*, I listed various categories of stress (with examples) that can affect you:

- **Environmental stress**—The sights, sounds, and smells around you in your home, workplace, your school, and your community

- **Physical stress**—Chronic pain, illness, surgery, and undergoing invasive diagnostic procedures

- **Emotional stress**—Anxiety, depression, despair, and PTSD

- **Spiritual stress**—Feelings of alienation, isolation, and challenges in one's spiritual faith

- **Pharmaceutical stress**—The negative side effects of many medications, as well as the related depletion of nutrients that can occur

- **Dietary stress**—Food allergies, adverse food reactivity, and nutritional deficiencies

- **COVID-19 pandemic stress**—This is a new one that everyone has struggled with in the past few years, which consists of the numerous stresses caused by the COVID-19 epidemic; these include frustration, feelings of isolation, disruption of daily routines, economic challenges, and coping with COVID symptoms

Stress can cause excessive inflammation in the body. Inflammation is helpful at first, because it is the body's way of fighting infection by increasing your temperature and causing swelling. But, like stress, inflammation that becomes chronic is harmful. Chronic inflammation increases pain and the breakdown of tissues in the body. Unchecked inflammation can also impair the immune system and render it less effective in protecting us from illness.

Excessive stress can even harm the DNA in our cells. Exposure to chronic stress and stress hormones such as cortisol can decrease the health and length of the protective casings at the ends of strands of DNA (telomeres). These casings are necessary for appropriate cell regeneration. As telomeres deteriorate, cells are impaired, or may become pro-inflammatory. This can increase chronic pain and accelerate the aging process.

Ultimately, poorly managed stress can maintain and worsen chronic pain. Stress commonly increases depression, anxiety, sleep disturbance, and relationship problems—all of which heighten the experience of pain. The chronic inflammation that is increased by stress renders nerve and muscle tissue more vulnerable to increased pain. Stress can increase dysregulation of your autonomic nervous system and heighten central sensitization, two of the big drivers of chronic pain.

Stress is a part of life—there's no avoiding it. That is why it is important to learn to recognize stress, observe it, and have strategies to respond to it.

For chronic pain sufferers, *stress* is anything but a neutral term. Most chronic pain patients have gone through a long, exhausting journey through multiple diagnostic tests with numerous health professionals who didn't solve their problem. When they hear the "S-word," many become very defensive, combative, or hopeless. *Stress* becomes a code word for "You're crazy," "Your pain isn't real," or "It's all in your head."

Let me reiterate a useful definition of stress for our purposes:

Stress is the perception that your capacity to cope has been exceeded.

Of course, the perception of stress varies widely for different people, as do the things they find to be stressful. We can illustrate this diversity by comparing the cases of two individuals who were treated in a pain center at a major metropolitan hospital.

Joe was a forty-seven-year-old narcotics officer. As a routine part of his job, he would raid crack houses. Every morning he would wake up, put on his bulletproof vest, and be ready to go. He had done this for so many years that he never even thought about it. No big deal. Until one day, when his squad raided a crack house...and Joe found his daughter there! At that moment, Joe's capacity to cope was exceeded. Soon after, his chronic low back pain flared up and Joe went to the pain clinic.

Cynthia was a fifty-eight-year-old multi-millionaire living in Southern California. She had significant symptoms of obsessive-compulsive disorder (OCD). She lived in an enormous mansion in Beverly Hills—so enormous that it had over 175 windows! Driven by her OCD, Cynthia was preoccupied with the cleanliness of these windows. She had all 175 of them professionally cleaned—every day! One week she decided to host a big party. And so, she had all the windows professionally cleaned, with extra emphasis to the cleaners to do an especially careful job, since there would be many guests. After the window cleaners left, and before the first guests arrived, a bird flew by and—*splat!*—it pooped on one of the freshly cleaned windows. That bird's dirty work exceeded Cynthia's capacity to cope. The thought of a party guest seeing that window caused a flare-up of her migraine headaches. They worsened in intensity and frequency, so she reported to the pain clinic.

Joe and Cynthia, two vastly different people, felt the effects of two vastly different kinds of stress. This shows how highly unique each individual's perception of stress can be. What these cases have in common is that there are two factors that determine the intensity of the stress—the *stressful event* itself and the *perception* of the event. Whether a tree falls on your car or you have a big argument with your supervisor, it's how you react to the event that determines its ultimate physiological impact. The same holds for your chronic pain, one of the major stressors in your life.

Please recall our discussion of the HPA axis (in the "Science of Chronic Pain" section) to get a reminder of how stress affects your brain and body. Your stress-response system does not care what caused the stress. It only responds to the intensity of your perception of stress, and then it automatically floods your body with stress hormones.

ONCE YOU'RE AWARE OF YOUR STRESSES, THEN WHAT?

Happily, many of the strategies you'll learn in the ABC method will help you with reducing the psychophysiological effects of stress. Virtually all the strategies listed in the next few chapters will help you fill your resource tank and will reduce the negative effects of stress.

CHAPTER 14

Awareness of Your Sleep

Chronic pain is one of the most common causes of insomnia. Up to two-thirds of all patients with chronic pain also experience sleep disorders. This causes a difficult vicious cycle: the pain interferes with healthy sleep, and sleep problems intensify the experience of pain. Autonomic dysregulation and arousal of the fight–flight response is very common in people who suffer from chronic pain, and is often a major contributor to sleep disturbance as well. Learning to calm this automatic response helps both to reduce chronic pain and to improve sleep.

Patients struggling with chronic pain face a Catch-22 conundrum when it comes to sleep disturbance. On one hand, we have ever-increasing scientific evidence of the necessity for everyone to get good sleep, and how poor sleep can lead to everything from immune deficiency and heightened risk of infections to cancer and stroke—not to mention chronic pain. On the other hand, we try to encourage our patients to take it easy when it comes to sleep. We teach our patients not to worry if they wake up, don't fight it. Not surprisingly, many of my patients tell me how they wake up in the middle of the night, and desperately try to get back to sleep because they are so worried about all the diseases that will befall them if they don't sleep!

Happily, there is a way to navigate through this confusing maze, and that is what we will address in this section. After exploring the relationship between chronic pain and sleep disturbance, we will look at the numerous contributors to the complex mix of insomnia and pain. Finally, I will share with you several strategies to heal your sleep.

Insomnia includes a range of sleeping problems, such as difficulty falling asleep, difficulty staying asleep, and waking up earlier than desired. In addition, many patients with chronic pain do not feel refreshed in the morning when they awaken, a problem called *non-rejuvenative* sleep.

Difficulty falling asleep is known in sleep medicine as *initial insomnia*. A common challenge for many with chronic pain is hyperarousal of the nervous system. When you are too stirred up and activated, it's difficult to drop your guard and let go of wakefulness in order to fall asleep. Furthermore, initial insomnia has its own enigma. Those of us who work in the sleep medicine field constantly teach our insomnia patients to make their bedrooms quiet and free of all possible distractions. Paradoxically, doing so may make the patient more aware of their painful sensations, thus interfering with falling asleep. Frequently, this leads to feelings of apprehension about going to bed, anticipating yet another struggle trying to fall asleep.

Another sleep problem is difficulty staying asleep, known as *middle insomnia*. That's when you fall asleep, but then wake up one or more times during the night. If you wake up at night and don't get back to sleep before it's time to get up, this is designated with the interesting and almost scary moniker *terminal insomnia*. Research shows that people with chronic pain may also experience several *microarousals* every hour. That means that you keep lapsing from deeper to lighter stages of sleep. Oftentimes it can be the experience of physical pain that causes the microarousal. Thus, chronic pain can cause a significant intrusion into a night's sleep and disrupt the normal stages of sleep.

Non-rejuvenative sleep—also known as non-restorative sleep—is diagnosed when the patient feels tired and sleepy during the day. This often occurs when people suffer with initial or middle insomnia. However, people who fall asleep well and do not awaken during the night can also experience non-rejuvenative sleep if they did not get enough deep-level sleep. It is common for chronic pain sufferers to have less efficient sleep— less deep sleep and more awakenings during the night. The quality of their sleep is often light—and not restful. Non-restorative sleep over an extended time can cause diminished energy, depressed mood, fatigue, and higher levels of perceived pain during the day.

Quality sleep is helpful for healing from chronic pain and for maintaining physical and emotional health. Good quality sleep protects against developing several types of health conditions. Better sleep improves cognitive functions such as memory, focusing attention, and concentration. Recent research suggests that during sleep a type of "rinsing" process takes place that cleans away waste products from the brain and central nervous system. This can improve and stabilize your mood. It can lower your risk for high blood pressure, heart disease, and stroke. Good sleep supports a healthy immune system and lowers the risk of developing certain types of cancer. It can lower your risk for developing diabetes and help you avoid unwanted weight gain.

As with any health condition, it is necessary to get a proper assessment of your sleep from a trained professional. If you have suffered with sleep disturbance for at least four weeks, it is time to get an evaluation from your primary physician or other sleep health professional. An assessment is also needed if you notice painful or agitated sensations when your legs have not been moving for a while—such as during sleep or during a long flight.

It is also necessary to seek professional assistance if you snore excessively or gasp for breath during the night. These behaviors raise the concern of possible obstructive sleep apnea. When apnea is present, a person's breathing is interrupted during sleep. People with untreated sleep apnea stop breathing repeatedly during their sleep, sometimes hundreds of times. This means the brain and the rest of the body may not get enough oxygen. There are two types of apnea, but the most common form is called obstructive sleep apnea (OSA). It is caused by blockage of the airway, usually when soft tissue in the back of the throat collapses during sleep. Factors that make apnea more likely include being overweight, having large tonsils, or a nasal obstruction due to sinus problems or a deviated septum. Common symptoms include loud snoring, daytime sleepiness, waking with a dry, sore throat, and recurring awakenings during sleep. If you have these symptoms, you should consider a polysomnogram, or a sleep apnea test. It takes physiological measurements while you sleep. The results are analyzed by a sleep specialist, who will then recommend treatment for OSA. The most common treatments include losing weight, treating allergies, a dental oral appliance to keep your airway open while you sleep, or a CPAP machine (continuous positive airway pressure) that keeps your airway open while you sleep.

Certain pain medications can interfere with healthy sleep. Opioids, for example—even after just a few doses—can contribute to sleep-related breathing problems, as well as disrupt sleep and prevent entering deep sleep. That is why you should report all your medications and supplements (both prescription and over-the-counter) when you are evaluated by your primary care provider or sleep specialist.

Another important factor affecting sleep is emotional distress. This includes anxiety, depression, or post-traumatic stress disorder (PTSD). Regardless of what type of emotional distress is present, one thing is clear: Sleep disturbance is one of the most common—and sensitive—indicators of unresolved emotional conflict. Sometimes the issues that we avoid or distract from during waking hours come home to roost when we no longer have external distractions—and bedtime is the most likely time for this to occur. In that case, availing yourself of brief psychological treatment may be helpful for addressing whatever is trying to get your attention during sleep hours.

WAYS TO HEAL YOUR SLEEP– TREATMENT OF CHRONIC PAIN– RELATED SLEEP DISTURBANCE

ELEVEN WAYS TO IMPROVE SLEEP HYGIENE

Just as good dental hygiene includes regular tooth brushing and good sanitary hygiene involves washing your hands, good sleep hygiene involves behaviors and practices that facilitate the best quality sleep.

1. **Preserve the sanctity of your bed.** Your bed should only be used for sleep and sex. It should not be a place for reading, watching television, or for struggling with falling or staying asleep. What does this mean?

If you wake during the night and cannot fall back asleep after twenty minutes, do not continue to try to get back to sleep in your bed. Instead, go to another room where you have arranged (in advance) to have a comfortable chair or couch. This dimly lit room is equipped with either music/headphones or a book with a clip–on light. The goal is not to *try* to get back to sleep, but rather to reduce struggle and just get comfortable. When you get drowsy, return to bed. If you don't get drowsy, at least you will reduce the struggle about getting to sleep, which helps to reduce overall agitation.

2. **Block off eight hours in your schedule for sleep.** Most people need at least seven to eight hours of sleep nightly to feel rested. So make sure that you have allowed at least this many hours in your schedule. For example, if your normal bedtime is eleven o'clock, make sure you don't have to get up until six or seven in the morning.

3. **Have a bedtime ritual.** Begin your ritual at least one hour before going to sleep. During this hour, ban all screens from the bedroom (television, computer, tablet, smartphone). Immerse yourself in a calming activity or non–news reading. During this wind–down hour, abstain from any complex problem–solving or relationship conversations.

4. **Find your natural time to go to bed.** When you are on vacation and not indebted to clocks and schedules, notice what appears to be your natural time to fall asleep. Once you have identified that time, stick to that time for going to bed on an ongoing basis.

5. **Maintain a consistent waking time.** Try as much as possible to wake up at the same time on weekdays as on weekend days. It is a myth to think that you can get by on four to five hours of sleep on weekdays and then binge–sleep for ten to twelve hours on the weekend. Over time this disrupts your circadian rhythm and leads to exhaustion and greater sleep difficulties.

6. **Prudent napping.** This is an interesting issue. Personally, I've never been a good napper—I would always emerge from the nap feeling somewhat drowsy. Some people I know can take a brief nap and wake

up refreshed. The evidence is mixed on whether napping interferes with nighttime sleep. My advice is this: Avoid daytime naps if you can. This will be best for supporting good nighttime sleep. If you must nap, keep it to twenty to twenty-five minutes, and no later than early afternoon. This will reduce interference with nighttime sleep.

7. **Do aerobic exercise earlier in the day.** Walking, biking, rowing, elliptical machine, or swimming can be very helpful for maintaining good sleep. Just make sure that your exercise ends by no later than four or five in the afternoon, so your body has time to wind down before bed.

8. **Watch your caffeine.** This stimulant can activate your sympathetic nervous system and interfere with sleep. If you do drink coffee or other caffeinated beverages, stop your daily consumption after lunch.

9. **Don't eat late.** It is best to allow at least two to three hours after your evening meal before bedtime. If your bedtime is at eleven o'clock, finish eating no later than eight or nine. If possible, refrain from any fluids for at least two hours before bedtime to avoid waking to use the bathroom during the night.

10. **Keep your bedroom cool, dark, and quiet.** Research tells us the optimum temperature for sleeping is anywhere between sixty and sixty-five degrees. Turn any clocks in your bedroom away from your view so that you don't check the time if you wake up.

11. **No pets allowed.** I know your beloved cat or dog is a member of the family, but your sleep comes first. It is best to keep your pet out of the bedroom overnight. Also, arrange to not be awakened by barking, clawing at the bedroom door, or having to wake up during the night to let your pet outside. This may take some negotiating with your spouse or family members, but a better rested, more pain-free pet owner will derive even greater joy from their furry friend!

IMPORTANCE OF CALMING TECHNIQUES
AND CLINICAL HYPNOSIS FOR SLEEP

It will help you sleep at night if you practice calming techniques often throughout the day. This will downregulate your internal idle speed and slightly lower the arousal level of your autonomic nervous system. Regular practice takes advantage of positive neuroplasticity to make a habit of this calmer mode of operation for your system. That will help your brain and nervous system be better prepared to downshift at day's end to calmness, quietness, and sleep. Use any of the techniques listed in the "Power of Breath" section of this chapter.

Add the daily practice of your twenty-minute self-hypnosis recording to your routine as well. Refer to the chapter titled "Clinical Hypnosis" in this book for more information. Hypnosis can also be used to specifically address sleep disturbance related to chronic pain. Ask your health provider for more information.

MEDICATIONS AND SUPPLEMENTS
FOR SLEEP DISTURBANCE

For some chronic pain patients, it may be useful to use a medication or supplement to serve as a temporary bridge for treating their sleep disturbance. There are many types of medication categories that may be recommended for this purpose. Here is a partial list:

- Analgesics such as acetaminophen.

- Non-steroidal anti-inflammatory drugs (NSAIDS) such as ibuprofen and naproxen.

- Muscle relaxants such as tizanidine, baclofen, cyclobenzaprine.

- Antiseizure medications (such as gabapentin, lamotrigine, pregabalin).

- Antidepressants (such as amitriptyline, trazodone, mirtazapine, duloxetine).

- Corticosteroids (including methylprednisolone—known as Medrol Dosepak—and prednisone).

- Benzodiazepines (such as lorazepam, clonazepam, diazepam).

- Prescription sleep medicines or "hypnotics" such as zolpidem (Ambien) or eszopicione (Lunesta).

- Over-the-counter sedating pain/sleep medications such as Tylenol PM.

- Herbal sleep supplements such as valerian root and melatonin.

These medications may be helpful in the short term as part of the treatment of insomnia in the chronic pain patient. In close communication with your specialist or primary care provider, you may choose to take one of these medications to get "unstuck." Remember, however, that from an integrative medicine orientation, it is wisest to view prescription medications as a "bridge" to where you can eventually call on your own self-healing resources to maintain your gains. You can read more about this in the chapter "Why Medications Don't Work as Well for Chronic Pain."

SLEEP HYGIENE WORKSHEET

What time do you go to bed? Is it the same time every night?

What time do you wake up in the morning? Is it consistent, or does the time fluctuate?

Do you tend to use your bed only for sleep and sex, or do you spend time in bed in the evenings reading, watching TV, and/ or looking at your phone or tablet?

How many hours of sleep do you need to feel rested? Do you allow for that number of hours in your sleep schedule?

How often in a week do you allow at least one hour of wind-down time before you go to bed?

_____

_____

_____

How often do you get aerobic exercise in a week? If you do exercise, what time is the exercise completed by?

_____

_____

_____

Over the past week, what time did you finish eating the last food? Drinking the last fluids?

_____

_____

_____

(Once you have answered these questions, look back over the last few pages of this chapter for guidance on what you are aiming for regarding these sleep hygiene skills.)

CHAPTER 15

Awareness of Your Diet

NUTRITION–PROVIDE YOUR CELLS THE RIGHT FUEL FOR HEALING

Recovery and restoration from chronic pain is a process achieved over time. As I mentioned earlier, it's like training for an athletic event. In rehabilitation as well as in athletics, your cells need the best type of fuel to support healing. Your muscles, nerves, and connective tissue need nutritional support during the process of strengthening, growing, and recalibrating.

In 2011, leading up to the release of my first book, *Trust Your Gut*, important discoveries were emerging in the medical literature about the *microbiome*, the ecosystem within the large and small intestine. It is home to many beneficial types of bacteria that affect digestion and other aspects of our well-being. The microbiome plays a major role in our immune response. Seventy-five percent of your body's immune receptors are located in the gut. It is also home to a majority of receptors for many important neurotransmitters, such as serotonin. What does this mean? Your gut microbiome is an important player affecting not only digestion but also your mood, your immune response, and even your chronic pain!

The gut microbiome plays a critical role in how much pain your body experiences. Recent research suggests that it deeply affects many types of chronic pain, including inflammatory pain, headache, neuropathic pain, and opioid tolerance.

INFLAMMATION AND CHRONIC PAIN

Inflammation is an important issue affecting your chronic pain, and the food you eat is a common source of inflammation. As I mentioned earlier, inflammation is the body's immune response to toxins as it works to cleanse itself. However, excessive inflammation triggers chronic conditions, such as chronic pain.

Many people are not aware that their diet can help prolong their chronic pain. Certain foods cause your microbiome to increase inflammation, which sends signals to your central nervous system that can promote chronic pain. The pro-inflammatory foods to be avoided include fried foods, sugary foods, and processed foods.

An anti-inflammatory diet may help reduce your pain. It can allow you to ultimately reduce the amount of medication you take. An anti-inflammatory diet can also reduce the unpleasant side effects of medications that cause brain fog, sleepiness, and memory loss.

THE MEDITERRANEAN DIET

The Mediterranean diet is a well-known anti-inflammatory diet. It was noted in the 1950s that heart disease was less common in countries bordering the Mediterranean Sea than it was in the United States. Since then there has been increasing interest in the traditional cuisines of Italy, Greece, and other countries in that region. Many studies have confirmed that the Mediterranean diet helps prevent heart disease as well as other chronic illnesses.

What kinds of foods are in the Mediterranean diet?

- **Beans:** black beans, kidney beans, chickpeas, navy beans

- **Nuts:** walnuts, almonds, pecans, cashews

- **Seeds:** sunflower seeds, pumpkin seeds

- **Plant foods:** peas and soy products, such as roasted soy nuts, edamame, and tofu

- **Whole grains:** brown rice, quinoa, whole-grain bread, oatmeal made from steel-cut oats

- **Fruits:** berries, apples, bananas, citrus

  Not fruit juice, since it often is high in sugar which is pro-inflammatory. Avocado is a good choice; it contains many beneficial nutrients and antioxidants as well as healthy monounsaturated fatty acids.

- **Vegetables:** dark, leafy greens, spinach, kale, broccoli, cauliflower, brussels sprouts, onions, cucumber, cabbage

- **Fish:** cold-water fish such as wild salmon, mackerel, rainbow trout, bass, tuna

  Farmed salmon is not healthy due to waste products and high levels of antibiotics.

- **Healthy oils:** extra virgin olive oil, which contains monounsaturated fatty acids and helpful antioxidants, as well as canola oil, avocado oil, and flax oil

- **Poultry:** chicken, turkey, pheasant

  Particularly white meat, removing skin when possible. Avoid frying, which is pro-inflammatory.

- **Lean red meat:** in moderation, especially grass-fed beef

- **Certain kinds of dairy:** low-fat yogurt, milk, and non-processed cheese

  Choose lactose-free milk if you have trouble digesting dairy.

- **Wine:** no more than one glass per day; red wine in particular may help to reduce inflammation

- **Tea:** green tea, black tea, herbal tea

- **Chocolate:** particularly dark chocolate with no less than 75 percent cocoa—no more than one ounce daily

Pro-inflammatory foods to minimize in your diet:

- White bread

- White rice, instant rice, rice and corn cereals, instant oatmeal

- Foods with high-fructose corn syrup (processed bakery goods, snack crackers, soda pop, and sweetened fruit juices)

- Processed meats (sausage, prepackaged lunch meats, bacon, and ham)

- Some oils and fats (shortening and margarine, and oils derived from corn, sunflower, or safflower)—trans fats in particular

INDIVIDUALIZE YOUR PAIN-REDUCING NUTRITION PLAN

Like all other advice in this book, your ABC healing plan works best when it is individualized for you in collaboration with the professionals on your healing team.

For more individualized advice when constructing your nutrition plan, be sure to consult with a registered dietician or nutritionist.

SECTION IV

Balancing

Introduction to Balancing

Try balancing on one foot. Notice that you sometimes start leaning in one direction, and in order not to fall, you must compensate by leaning in the opposite direction. If you had stayed still, you would have fallen. Maintaining balance is about recognizing you are getting out of balance and then righting yourself. Constantly.

Balance has been a vitally important concept in medicine and healing since the time of Hippocrates more than two thousand years ago. Hippocrates, the ancient Greek known as the "Father of Western Medicine," wrote how health and healing were dependent on balance. His philosophy held that maintaining health and fighting illness depended on natural elements. Beyond biology, health and disease are also affected by one's physical and social environment. Hippocrates wrote about the importance of maintaining equilibrium between all those elements of life over which we have some control. That includes one's relationship with air and water, food and drink, activity and rest, sleep and wakefulness, emotions and thoughts, and even the elimination of bodily waste.

Part of noticing you're getting out of balance is feeling exhaustion or grumpiness. Another indicator you're getting out of balance is feeling an increase in your chronic headache, rheumatoid arthritis, or chronic low back pain.

The equilibrium of our bodies is maintained by automatic processes that constantly self-adjust. Consider how our body's normal temperature is always around 98.6 degrees Fahrenheit. When we get overheated, we start sweating. The sweat evaporates and cools the body. When we are chilled, we sweat less and the blood circulation to the skin decreases. Any change that raises or lowers normal temperature automatically triggers an opposite, counteracting response.

If the imbalances increase too much, the counterbalancing mechanisms start to malfunction. If a person's body temperature shoots up above 107 degrees, the increased temperature speeds up chemical reactions that can raise the temperature even more. This imbalance becomes a vicious cycle that can cause severe illness or death if not corrected.

Our miraculous bodies are full of amazing examples of balancing. Make a fist to tighten your bicep muscle, and the triceps muscle on the back of your arm elongates and relaxes. Engage your core abdominal muscles and the muscles in your lower back start to relax. When you have an infection, killer T cells travel to the site of the infection to initiate an immune response to reduce infection. This is followed by suppressor T cells that ensure the immune response doesn't cause excessive inflammation. In our autonomic nervous system (ANS), the sympathetic branch triggers the release of fight–or–flight hormones to help us deal with threats of all kinds. The parasympathetic branch triggers the release of other hormones to calm down after the arousal is no longer needed. Our health depends on the countless acts of balancing.

Similarly, healing from chronic pain requires balance on multiple levels: Balancing the nervous system between activation and calming, balancing activity and rest (i.e., pacing), balancing needs for social support and alone time, and so on.

Sometimes maintaining balance can be challenging, even messy. Sometimes when we are overloaded and seek balance, we know we need to cut back but we can't cut back right away. We know we can't be balanced right now, but pledge to work toward restoring balance soon.

The centrality of balance in the human mind–body system makes it a key component of the ABC method for healing chronic pain. In the sections that follow, we will address some of the important aspects of balance and ways to achieve it.

CHAPTER 16

Techniques for Grounding, Calming, Balancing

FROM OVERWHELMED TO GROUNDED

Susan, a patient of mine suffering from fibromyalgia, described a typical day when her pain flares up: "Sometimes I have a day when my fibromyalgia manifests as a deep, aching pain in my neck and shoulders. It feels like no matter what I do to alleviate it, it hangs on stubbornly. After a number of hours, I feel consumed by this pain. There is now a level of muscle tension throughout my upper body. I want to go outside and walk but I hurt too badly, and besides, this pain is exhausting me. After a while, I feel so discouraged, so bitter. I can't look forward to any activities because it feels too overwhelming and hopeless. My thoughts are monopolized by worries and pessimistic preoccupation about how dismal my future looks. The more I try to change how I feel, the more stuck I become."

Many patients with chronic pain describe experiences like this. They feel like the pain takes over, dominating their thoughts, feelings, and sensations. If you ever feel this way, you can recognize the need for strategies to help you shake loose from the negative spell that the pain seems to be casting over you.

This is where grounding techniques come in. A grounding technique is a strategy to regain your balance by getting unstuck from patterns of negative emotional or physical states. They can help free you from panic, despair, pain-related tension, dissociation, and more. They work by pulling you back into sensory awareness of the present moment by focusing the mind in an easy, benign manner. A grounding technique does not delve into one's emotional experience or struggles. Instead, it is a way to coax yourself back into the present, rather than to be trapped with regrets about the past or anxieties about the future.

HOW TO GET GROUNDED

You may find it helpful to use the timer on your smartphone for this exercise.

1. Settle into a comfortable chair someplace where you will not be distracted for at least five minutes. (Indoors or outdoors)

2. After you sit down, rate the level of your tension/agitation on our 0–10 scale.

3. Take three slow deep breaths and settle more comfortably into that chair.

4. For the next two minutes, look around at everything that surrounds you. Focus only on the visual details. See how many different visual details you can notice. For each one, describe to yourself what you see. Verbalize it like this: "Now I see the green color of leaves on that plant." "Now I see the brown color of the wood on the side of the bookcase."

5. Focus strictly on the sounds around you for the next two minutes. Talk to yourself about what you hear: "Now I hear the sound of the ventilation system overhead." "Now I hear birds chirping outside my window."

6. For the next two minutes, focus strictly on the sensations in your body as you sit. Keep up the dialogue with yourself: "Now I feel the sensation of my left forearm resting on the arm of the chair." "Now I feel the sensation of my right foot on the floor."

7. After you have completed the above–mentioned steps, take another two or three slow deep breaths.

8. The final step is to return to where you started. Check your tension/ agitation level and rate it on the same 0   10 scale.

Susan, the patient above who was overwhelmed with pain and worry, tried out the grounding technique. This is what she said about it:

"When Dr. Weisberg first asked me to do the grounding technique, I was frankly annoyed. I was thinking 'I'm in real distress here and he's asking me to look at the bookcase?' At any rate, I allowed myself to notice sights—the lamp, the wooden desk, a rose color on a painting. By the time I got to noticing the sounds of cars driving by on the street, I noticed that I was already feeling a little calmer, and my neck pain wasn't making me quite as aggravated. By the end of the exercise, I not only felt calmness, but wasn't feeling as angry and hopeless about my pain flare. I wanted to keep doing the grounding for another ten minutes."

There are variations of this grounding technique that you might want to try:

- Place a cool or warm washcloth on your face and closely notice the sensation.

- Pick up a favorite book and slowly read the first two or three paragraphs out loud. As you do so, listen to the intonation of your voice.

- Walk outside or down a long corridor. Pay close attention to the sensation of each foot as it contacts the ground. Say "left" and "right" as each foot contacts the ground.

- Pick a category of objects and then think of as many items as possible that fit in that grouping. For example: How many states can you name? How many breeds of dogs can you name? Name the concerts you have attended.

- Take slow deep breaths for three minutes, focusing exclusively on the sensations of the breath in various parts of your body.

- Try walking barefoot outside on the grass or dirt. Pay close attention to the sensations of contacting the ground. Research suggests that walking barefoot can create added benefits of calming and pain reduction.

These brief exercises sound simple, but they can be very effective. It's surprising to be reminded how powerful a tool for comfort this can be. Grounding brings your mind and body into the present moment and is effective for getting "unhooked" from negative sensations, thoughts, and emotions.

Use any of the grounding techniques described above for at least five minutes. Then, describe what you notice feels different, both emotionally as well as in bodily sensations.

CHAPTER 17

The Power of Breath

"As newborns we enter the world by inhaling and when we leave at life's end we exhale."

—Christophe Andre, in *Scientific American*

Breathing is so identified with life itself that it plays an important role in many cultures and religions around the world. And for at least three thousand years, sages and healers have recognized that controlling the breath can improve health and well-being. The earliest traditions of yoga in ancient India were built around controlling breathing to increase longevity.

The primary purpose of breathing is to exchange gases in our body. Breathing brings in oxygen for our cells, and then carries away the waste product, carbon dioxide. Your breathing pattern changes when you are in pain or under stress. Your breaths become small and shallow. Shallow breathing, especially with rapid breaths (hyperventilation), can prolong your discomfort. It actually worsens the physical manifestations of stress and pain.

That's because breathing has the power to instantly change your nervous system. There are two parts of your nervous system, the part you control and the part you don't. You control the somatic nervous system, the part that activates the muscles that we can voluntarily move. You can raise your arm, scratch your nose, or clench your fist. The part you don't control is the autonomic nervous system. It is involuntary. It automatically regulates the functions of your bodily organs and their responses. If you become embarrassed, you blush. If you smell something delicious on the grill, you salivate. These things are involuntary.

Interestingly, breathing is the big exception to the rule. It is both voluntary and involuntary. Most of the time breathing happens automatically, especially when we are sleeping. But when we want to control it, we can. Go ahead and take a deep breath. Our voluntary control over the breath gives us a way to modify the autonomic nervous system and central nervous system—parts that are otherwise outside of our control.

The ancient wisdom of the power of breathing is now being scientifically supported by an increasing body of research. Studies on the physiological effects of modified breathing are showing a wide range of benefits. Breathing exercises can increase oxygenation, improve blood circulation, and lower blood pressure. It can also increase heart rate variability, an important measure of the balance and health of your autonomic nervous system. Breathing can improve the functioning of your immune system by reducing the levels of stress hormones in your system. Ultimately it can bring a feeling of increased physical energy and enhanced feelings of calm and well-being.

WHY IS BREATHING IMPORTANT FOR RELIEVING PAIN?

How can something as simple as a breathing technique have such a powerful effect on physical and emotional distress?

When you take a deep breath and exhale, the "magic" happens in part because the exhalation activates the vagus nerve. The vagus is the longest of the cranial nerves, extending from the head down to the abdomen. It is also highly connected to the function of the parasympathetic branch of the autonomic nervous system, the part that calms you down. An activated vagus nerve prompts the parasympathetic system to decrease alertness, lower blood pressure, and reduce the heart rate, thereby increasing calmness. This is one of the central physical correlates of the relaxation response. Understanding this helps to explain the effectiveness of Lamaze breathing techniques. They have been used over the last half-century by expectant mothers to reduce the pain and anxiety of labor and childbirth.

There is a powerful relationship between breathing and various physical and emotional responses. This is evident when I observe patients with breathing difficulties. It is estimated that about 60 percent of those with COPD (chronic obstructive pulmonary disease) have anxiety or depressive disorders. This is likely due to multiple contributing factors. We know that breathing in a shallow, faster pattern can decrease the quality of the oxygen supply and aggravate physical discomfort and anxiety. Breathing disturbances often trigger anxiety and even panic attacks.

The link between breath and emotional responses can be seen in those situations when you are on the verge of tears, and you don't want anyone to know. Remember our discussion about how emotions can only be experienced in the body? When you try not to show your grief, you instinctively constrict the muscles in your face, neck, and torso. Importantly, this includes tightening the diaphragm, the large dome-shaped muscle that separates your chest from your abdominal cavity. This is the major muscle for breathing. It contracts and expands rhythmically and continually—usually involuntarily. When you contract your diaphragm, it follows that your breathing becomes shallower, and you begin to feel progressively more uncomfortable. Likewise, we tend to instinctively hold our breath when we feel anxious or sad. And when we are experiencing pain, we tend to breathe in a shallow fashion and tighten and brace whatever area hurts. This is a good example of how the word *feel* applies both to sensations and emotions. When we are trying to not hurt so badly, we tighten our muscles and constrict our breath as the physical correlate of getting away from the pain.

Conversely, when you take deeper breaths, it is more likely that you will more fully feel whatever emotion may be residing within you. This almost always proves to be helpful in resolving difficult emotions. Similarly, breath techniques can also reduce the intensity and intrusiveness of physical pain.

BASIC BREATHING TECHNIQUES

For maximum effectiveness, find a quiet, relaxed environment where you won't be disturbed for at least five to ten minutes. Also, to notice the change that occurs, be sure to rate the level of tension/agitation that you feel on a 0–10 scale before you start the exercise, and then again after you finish.

DIAPHRAGMATIC BREATHING

This is a good, basic technique to introduce you to the benefits of mindful breathing.

1. Either lie down or sit up comfortably.

2. Place one hand on your chest and the other on your abdomen. Notice that your chest and abdomen are moving while you breathe.

3. Concentrate on your breath and try to breathe in and out gently through your nose. Your chest and stomach should be still, allowing the diaphragm to work more efficiently. Eventually you will feel your abdomen begin to rise with each breath, while your chest rises less.

4. With each breath, allow any tension in your body or mind to slip away.

5. When you have done this for three to five minutes, sit quietly and enjoy the sensation of physical and mental relaxation.

Now, take three to five minutes to practice diaphragmatic breathing. Describe below what you experienced after doing this, such as a difference in sensations in various parts of your body.

4-4-8 BREATHING

In this exercise you will learn to combine the physiological benefits of slow, deep breathing with the mind-quieting benefits of focusing on a target—in this case, numbers. The synergy that results is greater than if you were to strictly do either the breathing or the counting alone.

1. Settle into a comfortable position, either sitting or lying down. Close your eyes.

2. Breathe in through your nose while counting to four.

3. Hold your breath for four counts.

4. Exhale through your mouth for eight counts.

5. Repeat this cycle of 4-4-8 for two minutes or longer.

As you do this, it is important that you keep your attention focused on the counting. For this exercise and all the other techniques here, if your mind gets distracted during the practice, then just keep bringing your attention back to the counting once more.

Take three to five minutes to practice 4-4-8 breathing. Describe below what you experienced after doing this, such as a difference in sensations in various parts of your body.

SOMATIC FOCUS BREATHING

In this exercise you will achieve a calmer, more comfortable state while focusing the sensations of breath in three parts of your body: your abdomen, your chest, and your nostrils.

1. Sit or lie down in a comfortable position and start breathing at your normal rate and rhythm. There is no need to breathe more deeply or change your breath in any way.

2. As you breathe, focus your attention specifically on your abdomen. See how closely you can notice the various sensations there as your abdomen expands on the inhale and deflates on the exhale. Pay attention in this way for sixty seconds.

3. Next, switch your attention to your chest, breathe normally, and notice the sensations similarly to what you did in step two, again for sixty seconds.

4. Next, switch your attention to the rim of your nostrils and pay attention for sixty seconds.

5. Now, choose the part of your body that was the easiest to focus on, whether abdomen, chest, or nostrils. For the next five minutes, refocus your attention closely on that spot. Again, if you get distracted, just gently guide your attention back to the physical sensations in your area of choice.

Take three to five minutes to practice somatic focus breathing. Describe below what you experienced after doing this, such as a difference in sensations in various parts of your body.

3O-TO-1 BREATHING

This exercise is another effective way to synergize the benefits of nervous system modulation and mental calming.

1. Start either sitting or lying down comfortably. Close your eyes.

2. Take a slow inhalation, and as you do, think the number 30.

3. Take a slow exhalation, and as you do, think the number 30.

4. Take a slow inhalation, and as you do, think the number 29.

5. Take a slow exhalation, and as you do, think the number 29.

6. Continue this pattern of slow inhalation and exhalation as instructed above, with the number 28 and counting down to 1.

Take three to five minutes to practice 30-to-1 breathing. Describe below what you experienced after doing this, such as a difference in sensations in various parts of your body.

CHAPTER 18

Activating Strategies for Regaining Balance

You are likely familiar with the symptoms of a fight–flight response. They include heightened muscle tension, increased heart rate, sweaty palms, the feeling of a tight band around your head, heightened jitteriness, and restlessness.

But sometimes, the stress of your chronic pain may manifest instead in the freeze response. Manifestations of a freeze response may include feelings of lethargy, exhaustion, and paralysis, as well as emotional numbness, flatness, and disconnection.

If you are experiencing a freeze response, you may need an activating strategy, rather than a calming technique, to regain balance. Here are two examples of how to do an activating strategy.

ACTIVATING STRATEGY ONE

1. Sit on a chair or couch with good posture, head erect, feeling your back supported by the back of the chair or couch.

2. Take slow, deep breaths. Keep your eyes wide open.

3. As you do this, notice various sensations in your body, including the feeling of your back against the chair, your hands in your lap, and your feet on the floor.

4. Continue this practice for at least three minutes.

5. When done, sit on a chair and notice how your body and mind feel differently than when you started.

ACTIVATING STRATEGY TWO

1. Go into a long hallway inside or a long stretch of sidewalk outside where you can walk uninterrupted for at least thirty to forty steps without stopping or turning.

2. Stand tall, with good posture and head erect.

3. Start walking, making sure to swing your arms easily by your sides. Be sure to take long, full breaths. As you continue to walk, focus your attention on the sensation of your feet on the floor or sidewalk as you step.

4. Continue this practice for at least four to five minutes.

5. When done, sit on a chair and notice how your body and mind feel differently than when you started.

CHAPTER 19

Pacing: Balancing Activity and Rest

PACE YOURSELF

A local establishment in my neighborhood has a sign in front that displays various inspirational phrases. They will have familiar sayings like, "An apple a day keeps the doctor away" or, "If you believe, you can accomplish great things." But last week the featured message really got my attention. It said, "I don't work until I'm tired—I work until the job is done."

While this may be a helpful message for kids who are learning to develop a good work ethic, this is exactly the wrong message for patients with chronic pain. Our culture so values hard work and productivity that it is a sign of dishonor or weakness to do anything less than "get the job done now." It's part of our cultural DNA to always work longer and harder, no matter what ill effect it has on our physical, emotional, and spiritual health. This stoic mentality is hazardous for the chronic pain sufferer, whose muscles, nervous system, and connective tissue are already taxed beyond their limits.

WHY DOES CHRONIC PAIN CAUSE PROBLEMS WITH PACING?

You have likely found that chronic pain has changed every aspect of your life. One of the most basic yet important ways this happens regards how you carry out your daily activities at home and work. Chronic pain often leads to profound changes in our approach to activity, which manifests in different ways.

Some people give up on activities to avoid pain. They'll skip things like physical exercises, self-care, errands, or interacting with family and friends. Why do they choose to remain inactive? Perhaps the tendency toward depression, hopelessness, or exhaustion puts them in a passive mood. Maybe they have a sense of themselves as fragile and are just being cautious. It could be they have lost interest in activities because their pain has become so front-and-center that it dominates their daily attention. They feel there is no room or energy left for activity. Others withdraw because they feel ashamed or embarrassed to be seen in public when their health is less than vibrant. For these people, it is not acceptable to be seen as anything less than 100 percent capable at all times.

Others may choose inactivity because they have learned to disconnect from the sensations of their body until their body has to protest in the form of a major pain flare.

Others respond to their pain in the opposite direction. They defiantly push through while ignoring how they feel. They want to prove that their pain isn't defeating them. Why does this happen? They fear the danger of a slippery slope if they slow down at all. Unless they keep pushing themselves, they believe they may end up becoming disabled or debilitated.

The fact is that having chronic pain requires you to pay attention to things that people without pain don't have to. The goal is to find a moderate path to activity, which means pacing yourself. You must avoid the extremes of doing too much or doing too little. Learning to pace yourself is centrally important because it allows you to stay active. Pacing reduces pain flares, allowing you to do more of what is important to you. By regulating your rate of activity, you can feel more in control of your life.

Researchers have pointed out that pacing has two main benefits. First, it conserves energy for activities that are most important to you. Second, by starting a particular activity at a reduced rate, it allows you to gradually increase your time of doing the activity.

How does pacing work? The goal is to find the amount of activity that you can do without experiencing a pain flare afterwards. That limit applies to all activities—walking, biking, lawn mowing, light housework, etc. This is a little tricky at first, because sometimes there is a time delay between activity and flare. The flare may occur anywhere from two to twenty-four hours after the activity. It is best to start slow and give yourself a day of rest afterward to note the response. When you find the right amount of flare-less activity, stick with that amount, three to four times weekly. After a week or two at that rate, you can moderately increase the activity time. For example, if you are walking fifteen minutes daily, try increasing that amount to twenty minutes, and be sure to apply the twenty-four-hour test before staying at that higher level. This reduces the chance of a pain flare while you build your strength and endurance. Pacing enables you to gradually and safely increase your ability to do daily activities and reduce disability.

THE DANGER OF FEELING GOOD

One of the most common causes of a pain flare is overdoing it on days when you feel less pain. It is human nature to want to do more than usual when you feel better. So, it is very important to stick to your schedule even though you are feeling unusually pain-free on a particular day. Avoid the temptation to increase activity levels too much too soon.

As you learn the art of pacing yourself, one of your greatest tools is practicing sensory awareness of your body. This stems from the common tendency of pain sufferers to disconnect from the sensations and emotions experienced in the body because, well, it hurts. You need to stay alert to this bad habit of somatic disconnection. I keep repeating the importance of connecting to sensations in the body because it is an essential empowerment skill for managing pain. My motto is, "You can't change it if you can't see it." You need to pay attention to your body because it always provides you with clues in advance of a flare-up. For example, if you have low back pain, the clues could be a little sense of tightness in the low back, a subtle fatigue in the upper legs, or a slightly elevated sense of general agitation. If you ignore these sensations, then your body will turn up the volume on the pain to get your attention.

When you *do* notice the subtle tightening that precedes a flare episode, you can take steps to prevent the flare. Perhaps stop the activity you're engaged in. Do a three-minute breathing technique. Take five minutes to gently practice some of your stretching exercises. And then congratulate yourself—you have taken an important step toward making the next pain flare less likely!

CHAPTER 20

Balancing Social Time and Alone Time

GET THE SUPPORT YOU NEED

The health benefits of good social support have been empirically established for several decades. Positive social support makes you feel safe and cared for. It can also bolster your sense of purpose and self-worth, because good social interaction involves you giving time to and caring for others.

When it comes to healing from chronic pain, research shows that good social support gives you a greater level of resilience, which is vital to the healing process. In fact, people with low levels of social support are twice as likely to experience musculoskeletal pain. Conversely, people with chronic pain who report high levels of social support experience less distress and less severe pain. The more the support, the better the adjustment, even when chronic pain is bothersome. The impact and intrusiveness of pain is reduced when you feel included in supportive relationships.

Good social support helps in healing from chronic pain in several ways. Many studies show that people engaged in constructive activities and relationships are more likely to exercise, eat properly, have lower rates of substance use, and benefit more from active self-care. Polyvagal theory (discussed in the "Science of Pain" section) tells us that feelings of social connection and safety allow us to respond more easily and calmly to the stresses produced by pain. Additionally, being engaged in positive social relationships helps to direct our attention toward others instead of obsessing about our own pain.

Support groups are a great source of positive social interaction. One participant in a chronic pain support group had this to say: "It's so helpful to have a place to share not only the grief and hardship, but also hope and encouragement. We're not trying to fix anybody—just trying to help people cope with the pain." The typical pain support group will discuss strategies for coping with pain, deal with the stages of grief, reduce feelings of isolation, and share helpful breathing and self-massage techniques.

Not all chronic pain groups are necessarily beneficial, though. One study showed that a strong predictor of increased fibromyalgia pain was if someone participated in a fibromyalgia support group! This doesn't mean that all fibromyalgia groups are unhelpful. The devil is in the details. Groups that focus on a victim mentality were correlated with increased pain over time. There seems to be something debilitating about the siege mindset: "Nobody else understands how bad we pain sufferers have it, so we need to stick together." Groups that helped to improve pain and disability focused on healthy support, open communication, and personal empowerment.

HOW TO ESTABLISH BETTER SOCIAL SUPPORT

In addition to finding a good chronic pain support group, here are some additional strategies for bolstering your support network:

- **Volunteer.** You will meet others who share your values and interests when you choose a cause that's important to you and get involved.

- **Join a fitness group or gym.** You may establish new friendships while you exercise.

- **Take a class.** Either in-person or online.

- **Check the internet.** There are many good sites for people going through the stress of chronic illness. Meetup.com is a good source for many interesting group activities. Just be sure to do your due diligence and get references before getting started.

RESOURCES FOR FINDING A CHRONIC
PAIN SUPPORT GROUP

- The Pain Connection

- National Fibromyalgia & Chronic Pain Association

- MyChronicPainTeam

- Chronic Pain Anonymous

- American Chronic Pain Association

- Your local hospital community outreach office

CHAPTER 21

Posture Yourself: Balancing Your Body in Space

I want to alert you to the importance of posture as well as muscle strengthening and flexibility. You can use this introductory information as you start to work with your physical therapist (PT) in coming up with a healing plan to move you forward.

The focus here is to establish physical balance in your body posture. This will allow you to gradually increase your level of physical activity with greater comfort. Place your emphasis on slow, steady progress in achieving one exercise at a time to improve function and healing from your chronic pain. Your PT will likely work with you on the following goals:

- **Posture:** develop awareness of proper posture

- **Strengthening:** exercises that build stronger muscle (e.g., wall push-ups or bicep curls)

- **Cardiovascular:** light to moderate aerobic exercises (e.g., walking, swimming, or bike riding)

Let's discuss each of these components in a little more detail.

POSTURE

Attention to proper posture is critical to improving chronic pain symptoms. It can affect mood, blood pressure, pulse, lung capacity, and the function of your muscles and connective tissue. Poor posture has been shown to strongly affect such chronic pain issues as tension and migraine headache, temporomandibular disorders, back pain, and fibromyalgia. Poor posture can lead to fatigue, muscle spasm, and increased chronic pain.

Your PT will likely teach you postural exercises for multiple goals. One goal is strengthening core stabilizer muscles. The other goal is increasing somatic awareness, so you can begin to sense when your body is out of proper postural position. The PT will also likely teach you similar exercises for activating your core (abdominal muscles) and walking with improved biomechanics.

Let's go through what a postural exercise might be like. For example, if you have chronic headache, neck or shoulder pain, or jaw pain, your PT might show you what is called the "neutral spine" position. This refers to the correct position of your head, neck, and torso, to allow for the least amount of stress and strain. It also means that the surrounding musculature of your head, neck, and back can remain "neutral," in other words, not having to engage in overworking to support your upper body. When you are in this position, it maintains the natural curves of your spine. Then, the goal is to develop and support the surrounding muscles so that they can firmly yet comfortably help you maintain this neutral spine position while engaging in your normal daily activities.

How can you experience this example of neutral spine? First, settle into a chair. Pull your belly button in just slightly, to engage your core muscles lightly, mindfully. One way of accomplishing this is to do a chin tuck.

- Settle into a chair.

- Pull your belly button in just slightly, to lightly engage your core muscles.

- Gently bring your shoulders back and down, almost as if you were trying to bring your shoulder blades together.

- Do a chin tuck. While keeping your face in a vertical position (not tilting either up or down), gently push your chin back toward your spine.

- Another way to establish proper head position is to imagine that you have a string suspended from the crown of your head, and that you are going to pull upwards on that string until you have reached full extension.

Once you have learned how to reach neutral spine, your PT will encourage you to remember it in two ways. One way is *sensory*—pay attention to how it feels when you are in this position. The second way is *sensory and visual*—look in the mirror once you have established neutral spine so that you can connect how it looks and feels. This will help you to practice and reach it more easily in the future. Your PT might show you other types of neutral spine exercises in addition to this one.

STRENGTHENING

In addition to posture, muscle strengthening is very important. Whenever there is pain, your core stabilizer muscles become weakened. They are responsible for keeping your head, neck, back, legs, and torso in the proper position.

Then, even if your pain is relieved, the core muscle groups may not have been strengthened. This is part of the reason why people with chronic pain are so fatigued and often relapse. For this reason, strength exercises help ensure that you can maintain your improvements over time.

However, while you work on strengthening, awareness of muscle tightening is equally important. We know that people routinely tighten up sore areas—it's natural to brace and guard against pain. When it comes to strengthening, the muscles must be relaxed before they can be strengthened. Otherwise, trying to strengthen a tight muscle causes it to spasm. This not only increases pain but interferes with the strengthening process. Muscle tension is closely connected to the level of arousal in your autonomic nervous system. Many pain patients know this daily experience of being constantly on guard. This creates both chronic tension and exhaustion, part of the vicious cycle of chronic pain. So, learning to be aware of feelings of tension is very important.

Finally, your PT will encourage you to engage in some ongoing aerobic exercise, starting out gently. Aerobic exercise such as walking, biking, swimming, or elliptical machine increases tissue healing, improves muscle strength and flexibility, reduces nervous system sensitivity, and increases your body's production of endorphins (natural painkilling substances). An additional option is to find a PT who specializes in warm-water movement (exercises in a warm pool), so you can experience exercise benefits with the reduced gravity-resistance of water. (Note: you will find more detailed information about how to get started with physical exercise for healing chronic pain in the "Cultivating" section.)

CARDIOVASCULAR

Cardiovascular fitness is vital to your overall health, and it also supports your healing from chronic pain. This helps to explain, in part, why the ability to walk increasing distances is a very important index of recovery from chronic pain. Your healing team will be invaluable in helping you set up and follow your particular, titrated fitness plan.

Your PT will review all these considerations with you and come up with an individualized plan to help you gain the strength, flexibility, fitness, and somatic awareness to support progress on your healing path.

SECTION FIVE

Cultivating

Introduction
to Cultivating

The final stage of the ABC method to healing chronic pain is Cultivating. The basis of the program is for you to carry out a variety of self-care practices that unleash and sustain your innate self-healing resources. These inherent resources within you do not activate by themselves, automatically. Rather, you need to *cultivate* these capacities to make them available for healing.

We have already discussed the basic truth that the underlying problems surrounding chronic pain cannot be best treated by medication. The good news is that activity and sleep activate the most powerful pain-relieving systems in the body, and non-drug self-care strategies are the best way to strengthen them. This is why many experts in the chronic pain treatment field agree: *Self-care is the foundation of successful chronic pain treatment.* My goal for you is to supercharge your ability to cultivate your self-healing resources, through solid information and time-tested self-care strategies.

SETTING AN INTENTION

The first step for cultivating your self-healing resources is setting your intention.

The root of the word intention" ties back to the Latin *intendiere,* which means "to turn one's attention toward something," or literally "to stretch." Interestingly, the same root is also the basis for the word "tendon" (stretchy fibrous tissue that attaches muscles to bone). Successful rehabilitation requires you to turn your attention to the need to *stretch* yourself both literally and figuratively. You literally will learn how to stretch your muscles properly for greater flexibility, and figuratively you must learn to stretch yourself out of your usual comfort zone, to acquire new skills to take even better care of yourself and your healing.

Setting an intention makes it more likely that whatever change you want to make will actually happen.

After treating thousands of patients with all kinds of chronic pain, I have noticed a key ingredient in those who achieve the best long–term results. Sufferers who are more successful have embraced the program of skills and practices and have internalized their self–care activities. The routine has become a habitual part of their daily lifestyle, like brushing your teeth. They set intentions and follow through with them. They have learned an essential fact: When it comes to developing successful habits, repetition wins the day.

"To become really good at anything, you have to practice and repeat, practice and repeat, until the technique becomes intuitive."

—Paulo Coelho, Brazilian author

Those that fare less well tend to practice self–care reluctantly. They perform their self–care activities inconsistently, begrudgingly, like checking an item off a to–do list.

Athletes are used to setting intentions and goals, no matter what sport they participate in—track and field, swimming, football, etc. They affirm to themselves, "I will run an additional thousand yards at least twice in the coming week." "I will do stretching exercises for at least twenty minutes after each workout for the coming week." By following through on such intentions, athletes achieve excellence.

Success in healing from chronic pain requires a similar commitment. So how do you go about setting an intention for your healing practices?

From my observations as a clinical health psychologist, any type of behavior change is much more likely when you tie your intentions to your underlying motivation. Keep in mind not only *what* change you want to make, but also *why* it is important to you to make this change.

For example:

- Rather than telling yourself, "I need to drink less coffee," try instead to say, "I intend to spend more time feeling comfortable and alert rather than jittery."

- Rather than, "I have to do a breathing technique three times a day," instead try, "I intend to spend more time enjoying the feeling of calmness and vitality."

- Rather than, "I must stop eating so much salt and sugar," try instead, "I intend to spend more time enjoying the feeling in my body when I feed it healthier food."

EXAMPLE OF HOW TO SET AN INTENTION

1. Name the intention (for example: "I intend to practice the 4-4-8 breathing technique three times a day").

2. Briefly write down the reason why this is important to you (for example, I want to practice this daily because I know it will calm my nervous system and make my pain get better with time).

3. Write the intention down somewhere you can refer to it easily (such as a daily journal or a Post-it note on your computer or refrigerator).

4. Set a reminder, such as a beep or alarm on your smartphone, to remind you to do your practice at the same time every day (for example, set an alarm or reminder on your iPhone or Android phone to go off daily at nine o'clock, two o'clock, and seven o'clock).

5. Then, about once weekly, take a moment to notice how good it feels to set an intention of importance to you and then to carry it through. This is a tangible, concrete act of treating yourself with respect and care.

Whatever intentions you set regarding your chronic pain progress, don't forget to use your healing team as a helpful resource. The members of your healing team will help you set more specific intentions for such goals as improving your mood, decreasing aches and pains, eating healthier, and staying consistent with physical and calming exercises.

An important part of setting intentions is to build in a reward system to provide positive reinforcement along the way. For example, when you follow through on walking at least twenty minutes per day for at least three times in a week, treat yourself with something enjoyable. Maybe it's going to a movie, taking a drive to a favorite spot, or planning a weekend getaway at a bed and breakfast.

Finally, take it easy on yourself as you work on setting and following through on your intentions. Some of the symptoms of chronic pain—including exhaustion, depression, restlessness, etc.—can in themselves make it hard to stay consistent with follow-through. A trip to the emergency room or a pain flare episode can make you forget the intention you have set. Whatever the reason for your lapse, when you don't quite meet your goal for the week, don't punish yourself. If you remain gentle, kind, and non-punitive, you will be much more likely to bounce back more quickly. Then you can get back on track for the coming week without the self-sabotage that happens when you're too hard on yourself.

YOUR RESOURCE TANK

The journey of healing has its ups and downs. Setbacks are common because chronic pain sufferers must contend with an entire constellation of symptoms. Aching, burning, tightness. Exhaustion and depletion.

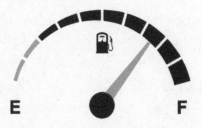

Difficulty falling asleep or staying asleep. Isolation from family and friends. Loss of interest in work and other daily activities. Little or no libido. The sluggishness that comes from no physical exercise over a sustained period. Feelings of anger, despair, desperation, futility, hopelessness. Loss of appetite.

But then there are times when things seem a little more bearable. The pain lets up a little. There's a little more energy, a little more interest in daily activities. Some return of libido. Glimpses of a little hope. Feeling your sense of humor return just a little. Sleep seems a little less elusive. Progress once again feels possible.

What determines whether you have an easier or tougher day? I've come to believe that a major factor is the state of your *resource tank*. Think of your resource tank as a gas tank. It's a reservoir of raw materials, the skills, tools, and energy needed to deal with and heal from pain. Patients with a full resource tank feel better and are far more able to cope well with the challenges of their pain. When your resource tank is running low, everything feels harder, more painful, more exhausting.

How do you fill your resource tank? Every time you practice the self-care strategies listed in this book, you make a deposit in your resource tank. Each new skill you master replenishes your reservoir of strength and confidence.

Every skill discussed in the chapters that follow in the "Cultivating" section of the book will help you make valuable deposits toward your resilience and long-term recovery.

Ready to start filling your resource tank? Let's begin.

CHAPTER 22

Limbic Retraining: Calming the False Alarm in Your Brain

So much of what you read and hear about in the pain treatment world is about how to get rid of and control pain. When you Google "What can I do for chronic pain?" you get a plethora of treatment recommendations. These include: all kinds of prescription and non-prescription pain medications; nerve blocks, spinal pain pumps, and spinal cord stimulators; trigger point injections; bioelectric therapy and TENS units; physical therapy; herbs; chiropractic; and more. All these treatments have the same goal: eliminate the pain, get the pain under control, get the pain to go away. All these modalities have merit and usefulness.

And, as I wrote about in my previous book on digestive distress called *Trust Your Gut*, much of our traditional Western medical approach to chronic pain involves violent war metaphors. Clinicians fight disease, wage war on chronic pain, and patients struggle valiantly to conquer the disease. The medical weapons arsenal includes lasers, radiation, chemicals, electricity, and pills. The primary goal is to kill the pain.

When chronic pain has caused such suffering and has turned your life upside-down, it's understandable that you would hate your pain.

IT'S NORMAL TO HATE
YOUR CHRONIC PAIN

This quote captures the feelings I hear conveyed by so many of my patients who suffer from chronic pain:

"I've struggled with chronic back and shoulder pain for ten years. On some days I can get up and go through my workday more or less unencumbered. But on some mornings, I just can't get out of bed no matter how hard I try. This is because I may awaken with headaches, body aches, shooting pains down my legs, and a feeling like I'm dragging a hundred-pound weight on my chest. This suffering is not only painful but also unpredictable. When my body has caused me so much suffering, how can you blame me for hating it? I hate it for holding me back from everything I want to do in life. I know I shouldn't feel this way—and then I hate myself for feeling this way."

LEARN TO BEFRIEND YOUR BODY

This may sound counterintuitive, but a key way to conquer your chronic pain is to quit fighting it. A nonviolent approach to healing certainly goes against the mainstream attitude toward illness. As we just reviewed, clinicians wage war on chronic pain, and patients struggle valiantly to defeat the disease. So much of what you read and hear about in the pain treatment world is about how to get rid of and control pain. The primary goal is to *kill* the pain, which is why *painkillers* are so often referred to.

This misguided attitude toward illness is fueled by the fact that people tend to hate their pain. This antagonism is quite understandable.

It's quite normal to hate your pain when it has caused so much suffering, so much disruption. It overwhelms you and leaves you feeling hopeless. If you feel like this sometimes, know that you are not alone.

It is also quite common to view pain as the enemy. It must be fought against at every turn until it is defeated. For if the pain is the enemy, then it must be defended against, braced against, guarded against. If there is an enemy in your midst, you must become hypervigilant against this ongoing threat.

While it is easy to understand why you hate your pain, you need to know that this response is counterproductive. If we look at how hate actually functions in your nervous system, we can see how it can worsen chronic pain.

WHAT HAPPENS PHYSICALLY WHEN YOU HATE YOUR PAIN

Several things happen physiologically when you hate your pain sensations. First, you wake up the *limbic system*, the threat–perception circuitry that resides in the deeper part of your brain. The limbic system is the security guard of the brain. Once it perceives a threat, it reacts by setting off an alarm telling the autonomic nervous system (ANS) to activate a fight/flight response. Your hate is interpreted by the brain as a threat, so it gears up the body to go into action—sensitizing your muscles and nerve channels. This makes your pain worse. Remember that your ANS is already dysregulated, a major cause of chronic pain in the first place. It suffers from an imbalance between the activating (sympathetic) and calming (parasympathetic) branches. Every time you feel a surge of hate toward your pain, the ANS becomes even more dysregulated—causing a vicious cycle. This is how hate increases your pain. Viewing pain as your enemy is counterproductive.

Hating your pain also backfires by increasing negative *pain conditioning*—like Pavlov's dog. Pavlov conditioned dogs to salivate when he rang a bell. He did this by ringing a bell every time the dogs ate. They initially salivated because of the food, but their bodies became conditioned to associate the bell with eating. After a while, the sound of the bell made them salivate.

Likewise, humans with chronic pain condition their nervous systems to overreact. Because chronic pain evokes such strong emotional responses, conditioned responses to pain happen all the time. For the chronic back pain or headache sufferer, pain conditioning can cause added distress that intensifies and maintains the symptoms. A twinge in the low back, cramping in the gut, or a deep dull ache in the forehead can lead to powerful conditioned reactions of anger, despair, anxiety, agitation—and even hatred. These conditioned emotional responses can create a cascade of physiological changes that maintain and worsen the pain.

Another physiological effect related to pain and conditioning is *state-dependent memory*. This is the phenomenon where one aspect of a terrible experience sparks a vivid flashback of the entire memory—like my friend who drilled through his finger. Now, every time he sees a drill, it makes his finger hurt. State-dependent memory occurs when some sensory aspect of an experience backs all the experiences associated with the original trauma. Your sensation of pain may have become part of a state-dependent memory that calls forth the emotions of hatred and agitation. This becomes another vicious cycle, where the current pain and agitation triggers a state-dependent memory of all the previous times when this suffering has occurred. This makes the pain much harder to treat.

When hating your pain becomes habitual, that habit is reinforced by negative *neuroplasticity*. As we discussed earlier, neuroplasticity is the capacity of the brain to build new neural connections in response to repetitive actions. When chronic pain becomes connected with feelings of hatred and agitation, new nerve patterns form in the brain. Going forward, the painful sensations get automatically connected with emotions of agitation and hate, every time.

GOING AWOL: DEALING WITH PAIN THROUGH DISSOCIATION

Yet another common reaction to the sensations of chronic pain is to escape by disconnecting from it. Often people distract themselves from it with other activities, including eating, drinking alcohol, or taking drugs. The clinical term for this is dissociation, which we discussed in Chapter 4, "Awareness." A popular method of distraction is to stare at a screen. You can watch television or a movie, play a game, or mindlessly surf the web. People learn to dissociate from the sensations of their body, cut their mind off from the discomfort—until it becomes so painful that they can't ignore it anymore.

With acute pain in the short term, this is a useful strategy that we all use. For example, when we bump our shoulder or elbow, we will sometimes rub the area. This provides a distraction by applying a competing sensation. But in chronic pain, dissociation can become a problem. A good example is the case of a former patient named Fred. He was a postal worker who had complex regional pain syndrome (CPRS) in his foot. Fred tried to cope with his pain by mentally dissociating his foot from the rest of his body. As a result, he started walking differently, keeping balance differently, and this ultimately made his pain much worse.

THE BETTER ALTERNATIVE: BEFRIEND YOUR BODY THROUGH LIMBIC RETRAINING

Although hating your pain is understandable, it causes a destabilizing effect on your nervous system and is guaranteed to make your pain worse. Instead of this harmful and counterproductive attitude, you need a way to pay attention to your pain sensations in a manner that is therapeutic and helpful. You need a more constructive mindset to respond to your symptoms, one that creates positive state–dependent memory and positive neuroplasticity. What's needed is for you to befriend your body, to become its ally. Healing becomes possible when you learn how to care for, appreciate, and show kindness to the sensations that have been plaguing you. That's where Limbic Retraining comes in.

Limbic Retraining is a powerful method for rewiring the pathways of nerves and hormones that are central to the physiological communication system that we call the *pain network*. This is a deceptively simple yet very effective tool for healing your chronic pain.

The key to Limbic Retraining is developing an attitude of curiosity, acceptance, and patience toward the pain sensations you are experiencing. This is the middle ground between fighting the pain and ignoring it. Instead, just notice it, observe it, and feel it. Allow the sensation to be there exactly as it is.

It may seem disorienting and a bit of a shock to reach out with kindness to an old foe.

Sid, a patient in his late forties with chronic arm and shoulder pain, was asked to experiment with sitting with the painful sensations in his hand and arm for just a short time. His response: "There is no way I will just notice that pain without trying everything in my power to fight it and defeat it! If I were to allow that pain to be there without trying to make it go away, then I am terrified that the pain will win and I will be rendered a powerless, defeated, hopeless victim."

I've had many patients like Sid who expressed an initial reluctance to do an about-face and try such a shockingly different approach. However, it is also shockingly effective and shockingly simple.

HOW TO DO LIMBIC RETRAINING

1. Sit in a comfortable and balanced position where you won't be disturbed for at least five to fifteen minutes.

2. Focus on the uncomfortable sensation in your body—the head, neck, back, gut, or wherever the pain is. If helpful, you can use your hands to help you visualize how large the area of distress is.

3. Rate the intensity of the discomfort on a 0–10 scale, where 10 is the worst pain you have ever experienced and 0 is no pain at all.

4. Now, on the same 0–10 scale, rate the *intrusiveness* of this pain sensation. In other words, how much does this pain interfere in your daily life right now? Is it just a mild irritant, or is it so front-and-center that it demands your complete and full attention to the exclusion of everything else?

5. Now, focus on the sensation *without thinking about it*. This exercise is calling on your *sensory attention*, not your ability to think. For example, imagine what it would feel like if somebody gently put their hand on your arm right now. Focus on the sensation exactly as it is, letting yourself be curious about it. I use the term *curiosity* here very intentionally. Curiosity implies steady, focused attention to something while staying calm and non-reactive. You can't be curious and anxious at the same time.

6. Imagine that you are going to pull a chair up right next to the sensation and just observe it exactly the way it is, without trying to change it, move it, analyze it, or make it go away. This would be a good time to remind yourself: "I may not like this sensation, but I'm remembering that it has been medically evaluated and that it is not going to harm me. So, for at least the next few minutes, I'm going to let it be there exactly the way it is and just observe it."

7. Now, give it time—as opposed to "I've done this for a minute—why isn't the pain gone yet?" As you sit with the sensation, you may feel compelled to *do something to fix it*—whether that means trying to relax it away with deep breathing, or visualizing it going away, please do not succumb to that impulse! Don't try to magically wish it away. This is the time to do a little twist on the adage, "Don't just do something—*sit* there!" By not trying to do anything, you activate natural self-healing resources. Just sit with it and observe—and let this be an interesting experiment as you learn a new response to an old and stubborn problem. By focusing and observing the sensation without trying to fight it, you are activating parts of the brain that are not associated with threat and guarding.

8. Stay with the cutting edge. Continue to stay focused on the part that either hurts the most, or most grabs your attention. And make room for whatever happens next. This means that, for example, you may start focusing on a deep pain in your left lower back, but then after a while it migrates to a lighter, tingling ache in the right lower back, and then to a mild ache in your middle back. By staying with this most dominant sensation wherever it leads, you will maximize

your inner healing resources for retraining the responses of your back, your nervous system, and your brain.

9. Remember—at times you may become so impatient or mad at the pain that you slip into fighting it once again. With practice, it will become easier to sit with it without struggle. Some patients have described this as "breaking through the wall"—just like the long-distance runner who feels out of breath and suddenly gets his second wind.

10. Sometimes the sensation may not change much, but you may end up getting a hunch or clue about something that is important to your healing. You may notice a revelation pop up, such as "I'm really upset at my spouse for not paying more attention to me." Or "I'm really exhausted and need some rest." Or "I'm in the wrong job—I really hate it." When hunches or clues such as these emerge, pay attention to them. They might lead to a redirection or lessening of the pain sensations once you heed the message.

11. Don't be surprised if Limbic Retraining feels challenging or awkward when you first start practicing. You are learning to change a natural reflex to avoid or struggle against pain. This often takes longer to learn than relaxation exercises or breathing techniques. After all, you are learning to counteract or re-do what has been a lifelong habit of fighting unpleasant sensations. With regular practice, you will be pleasantly surprised to notice how the practice becomes easier, and how you can enjoy learning to listen to the wisdom of your body as you stop fighting and hating it!

12. Repeat this process whenever your pain sensations become bothersome.

Now, why is that so important?

This exercise sends signals to structures deep inside your limbic brain. In a language they can understand, you are saying to the amygdala and related limbic brain structures: "This sensation that alarms you is actually no longer a threat." As you repeat this exercise, the limbic brain starts to signal to the nervous system and hormonal system that these sensations of pain, ache, and pressure are actually not a cause for alarm. Over time this causes a change in the cascade of neurotransmitters and neurohormones that communicate with these painful parts of your body. You are establishing new patterns of positive conditioning and positive neuroplasticity. My patients are almost always amazed to discover how much their pain sensations move, change, and quiet down with Limbic Retraining.

BENEFITS OF LIMBIC RETRAINING

Limbic Retraining helps you, the pain sufferer, to experience a very powerful and important message:

This symptom can change, and the intensity is temporary.

Other benefits from this practice continue afterward: 1) You start to remember and believe in the changeability of symptoms. 2) You can remember at other times, "These sensations are a nuisance, but they're not going to harm me."

Marcie is a twenty-six-year-old student who also worked part-time in an IT (information technology) firm doing web design. She presented to my office with severe left-sided neck and shoulder pain of three years duration. She described her neck and shoulders as "rock hard" and that every time she turned her head, she felt sharp stabbing pain that radiated from her neck and shoulders, down her back, along her spine, 7 to 8 out of 10. By the time she came to me, three years after diagnosis, Marcie felt increasingly irritable and distracted by her pain. She had also developed a headache resulting from the chronic neck and shoulder tightness.

She worked with me to learn about her chronic pain. She also learned a number of calming techniques and the "Neutral Spine" posture to more fully support the weight of her head and neck on her shoulders and back.

When introduced to Limbic Retraining, Marcie's first response was, "Accept the sensations being there? After all the grief and misery it has caused me? I'd have to be crazy to do something like that!"

Eventually, since none of her other coping strategies were working, Marcie reluctantly agreed to focus on the outer edge of her tight, sore neck and shoulders. At first, she still tried to force it away. Then, she finally stopped fighting it and allowed herself to simply feel the ache and tightness. After about five minutes, her eyes began to well up with tears. "The achy tightness is almost gone. How can that be?"

I explained to her that her nervous system needed her to stop fighting the symptoms and begin to befriend and listen to them. Marcie recognized she was experiencing tears of joy because there was now hope that these stubborn symptoms could finally begin to change.

CHAPTER 23

Clinical Hypnosis: Cultivating Your Brain for Healing

"The voice talking to you gradually becomes more distant, and you find yourself forgetting that it is there...but somehow the soothing voice continues to affect you, gently and almost automatically."

—Dr. Olafur Palsson, Clinical Psychologist, University of North Carolina

My patients are always eager to hear about one of my favored techniques, a powerful tool that I recommend for chronic pain. I tell them it is a perfectly natural therapy that is remarkably effective with virtually no negative side effects. Research has shown it can reduce the intensity, duration, frequency, and intrusiveness of chronic pain. It is beneficial for a multitude of chronic pain conditions (including cancer, low back pain, headache, neck pain, arthritis, temporomandibular disorders, burns, sickle cell disease, fibromyalgia, complex regional pain syndrome, and physical disabilities).

Whew! What is this medical marvel?

That's when I break the spell and tell them, "It's clinical hypnosis." Their eyes drop a bit, and they lean back in their chair. You don't have to be an expert in body language to realize they are a little apprehensive about the idea of being hypnotized. I've seen this reaction many times, and the story is always the same. They generally have no idea of what clinical hypnosis really is. Their understanding of hypnotism usually is based on what they have seen in movies and on TV. And like everything else that comes out of Hollywood, it is long on entertainment value and short on truth.

They picture Svengali or Count Dracula, who seize control of the minds of beautiful maidens with a mesmerizing stare and a simple command: "Look into my eyes!" Other popular images are a pocket watch on a chain swinging back and forth, or a spiral disc that rotates to hypnotic effect. "You are feeling sleepy⋯" In a fan-favorite movie, it is the recurrent sound of a spoon stirring a cup of tea.

Regardless of how the hypnosis is induced, the effect is always the same. The subjects fall into a trance and their minds are reprogrammed by the hypnotist to carry out evil deeds against their will. When the subjects wake up, they don't remember any of it. Sounds scary, doesn't it?

Yes, this sort of hypnosis is a great plot device, but it is complete hogwash.

This is where I launch into my spiel about all the things that are wrong with this view of hypnosis.

THE FIVE FALLACIES OF THE HOLLYWOOD HYPNOSIS HOAX

Fallacy One: When you snap out of a hypnotic state, you won't remember anything.

Fact: People generally remember most of what happened while they were hypnotized. Amnesia during hypnosis is very rare.

Fallacy Two: You can be hypnotized against your will and lose control over your actions.

Fact: Hypnosis works best when the patient voluntarily participates in the treatment. Many studies have shown that the patient cannot be hypnotized into doing something against their will or value system.

Fallacy Three: Hypnosis will make you lose consciousness.

Fact: Numerous EEG studies have demonstrated that hypnosis is not sleep. Most often, the patient will be conscious of everything going on while in the hypnotic state. However, sometimes you may relax so much during hypnosis that you drift off and lose track of what is happening. And if you are sleep-deprived, you might even fall asleep from the deep relaxation!

Fallacy Four: Hypnosis will force you to reveal secrets about yourself.

Fact: As mentioned above, hypnosis will not cause you to do or say things against your will. Hypnosis during psychotherapy may sometimes be used to explore unconscious material, but this is only done with the mutual consent of patient and doctor. When hypnosis is used for relief of a physical problem such as chronic pain, no such uncovering is typically needed.

Fallacy Five: People who can be hypnotized are more gullible or simpleminded.

Fact: Wrong! If anything, the capacity to experience hypnosis correlates more with openness to new experiences, rather than gullibility.

That other branch of show business that uses hypnosis for the sake of entertainment—stage hypnosis—is largely built on these same fallacies. You may have attended a convention or party where they hired a stage hypnotist. This is someone who is not a health professional, but has learned enough to put somebody into a trance. I can understand how people may enjoy watching a group of volunteers from the audience start barking like dogs. But this is a distortion of what hypnosis is. Worse yet, when your first exposure to hypnosis is riddled with fallacies, it is hard to take it seriously as a safe and useful treatment for distress.

NATURAL HYPNOSIS

The great irony of hypnosis is that it seems like such a mystery, yet we naturally enter hypnotic states every day:

- When you daydream during an activity

- When you get so involved in a hobby or other activity that you lose track of time

- When you watch a movie or TV

Experts in hypnosis have identified three basic features that characterize the genuine hypnotic state: dissociation, absorption, and suggestibility. You are likely to be familiar with all three.

1. **Dissociation**—We've discussed dissociation previously as a coping technique of disconnecting with pain by ignoring sensations. Basically, any kind of disconnection with what is happening in us and around us is dissociation. It is what you mean when you say someone is "spaced out." They are in their own world and are not paying attention to anything outside it. It's like that time you were driving home from work and started wondering about what was going to happen next on *The Crown*. You started reviewing in your mind all the key scenes from last season. You're in the middle of a great scene—when suddenly you are forced to stop daydreaming because you find yourself pulling into the driveway in front of your house! You had no memory of all the turns and roads you took to get home. You were spaced out. You were dissociated. You were hypnotized! Under this kind of natural spell, people commonly lose track of time. And they frequently report having a floating sensation, which makes sense because they certainly aren't grounded.

2. **Absorption.** Being absorbed in something you are doing is an act of full concentration. Absorption is being totally immersed in an activity. People say they are "in the zone" or "in the flow." A jazz artist might say he is "in the groove." When you are totally focused

on your activity—whether it is gardening, making music, or playing sports—you are oblivious to everything else going on in the world. Another way of saying it is that nothing distracts you. The NFL quarterback in the final seconds of a tight game pays no attention to the deafening crowd noise. Anyone seriously involved in a hobby knows this state. Think of how time flies and you become totally engaged in cooking, reading, painting, or gardening.

You are in a similar absorbed state when you watch a movie or a play—you suspend disbelief and forget about the outside world. That's why you hate it so much when someone starts talking in the theater—it breaks the spell. That's also why you can binge-watch a TV series and have no clue as to how many hours you just wasted. It also explains why some people can't stop playing video games. That could be considered the downside of this naturally occurring hypnotic state. But for those who are practicing their craft, there is nothing more desirable than being "in the zone."

3. **Suggestibility.** It is a feature of the hypnotic state that a person's mind has a heightened openness to suggestions. An everyday example is when the mother kisses away her child's boo-boo, and makes the pain go away. When the toddler falls and scrapes her knee, she starts crying with all her might. But when Mommy reassures her and kisses the injury, the pain goes away, the crying stops, and the little girl smiles. The mother's gesture changed her child's perception of pain. This phenomenon works for adults, too, which is why many clinicians use hypnosis to treat chronic pain. It is this same openness that makes hypnosis a door to the mind and body where positive suggestions can enter.

A common feature that runs through all these aspects of hypnosis is a distorted sense of time. When you are sitting through a boring lecture or a dull meeting, it feels like time is standing still. The clock moves so slowly you think the event will never end. But when you're on a great vacation, time speeds by and it's all over before you know it. It is common for people to underestimate the length of time they have been hypnotized.

CLINICAL HYPNOSIS

Clinical hypnosis is where a trained health professional induces a hypnotic state and uses therapeutic suggestions with a patient, primarily with the goal of relieving pain or suffering. One definition of hypnosis comes from the American Psychological Association: "A set of techniques designed to enhance concentration, minimize one's usual distractions, and heighten responsiveness to suggestions to alter one's thoughts, feelings, behavior, and physiological state."

In this way, clinical hypnosis methodically makes use of the features of natural hypnosis—dissociation, absorption, and suggestibility—to serve a broader therapeutic purpose.

It is important to emphasize that clinical hypnosis is not a treatment in and of itself. Rather, it is a procedure that can be used to facilitate other types of therapies and treatments. For example, hypnosis is not a type of psychotherapy, but it is a technique that can enhance the effectiveness of psychotherapy.

People commonly confuse hypnosis with meditation. There are similarities between them, but their differences are important. Both are beneficial forms of focused awareness that usually bring a feeling of calmness and relaxation. However, relaxation may not always be a goal of hypnosis. Such is the case with *active-alert hypnosis*, a method used by athletes, test-takers, and others to maintain focused attention during activity to enhance performance. Another primary difference between hypnosis and meditation is the goal of each practice. In meditation, the goal is to enhance nonreactivity of the mind, which may reduce stress levels and ultimately calm the body. Both hypnosis and meditation are worthwhile practices that are helpful for healing from chronic pain. In hypnosis, the goal is to take advantage of this receptive state to offer specific *therapeutic suggestions* to create changes in your thoughts, emotions, and physiology.

THE IMPORTANCE OF SUGGESTIONS

Hypnotic suggestions can effectively change certain ways that your body/ mind functions. During hypnosis, I will offer a suggestion designed for a specific patient. For example, I may say, "You will find that the tight constriction around your head will start to loosen" or "You'll be pleasantly surprised to notice yourself falling asleep at night much more easily and waking up refreshed and rested." Notice that these suggestions can either have an immediate effect, or instill positive inclinations for the future. The remarkable thing about suggestions made during this receptive state is the effect they have on autonomic (that is, automatic) processes. Suggestions give you the ability to rewrite your inner narrative. It is an effective way to begin to root out negative habits by replacing them with positive ones. Self-hypnosis can be viewed as the ultimate act of self-control. It allows people to change the way they feel and to use more of their potential.

Other hypnotic suggestions can be used to bring healing and relief. In a state of concentrated attention, ideas and suggestions that are compatible with the patient's desires can have a powerful effect on mind and body. For example, a patient with low back pain may be given a suggestion to picture being able to move, sit, and bend in the future while feeling increasingly comfortable and confident in his body's ability to heal from back distress.

Practitioners conduct clinical hypnosis in different ways, but virtually all encourage the use of the imagination. Mental imagery can be very powerful in a state of focused attention. For example, a patient with a chronic muscle tension headache may be asked to imagine what her distressed head feels like. If she imagines it as a constricting belt around her forehead that is being continually tightened, I can suggest she imagines the belt is being gradually loosened and her forehead is becoming more relaxed and comfortable. Activating the imagination can yield beneficial physiological changes.

HOW DOES HYPNOSIS WORK
FOR TREATING CHRONIC PAIN?

Research has established that hypnosis can be a powerful way to change the way we use our mind to enable new physical and emotional responses. We are also seeing studies that attempt to track what is going on in the brain and nervous system during hypnosis. We are still in the early stages of mapping out the neurophysiology of hypnosis, but we are developing some useful hypotheses that give us an idea of what is going on.

One main tool in such research is fMRI—functional magnetic resonance imaging. Images captured during hypnosis indicate that some areas of the brain become more active and other places become less active. As I discussed earlier, patients with chronic pain commonly suffer from dysregulation of the autonomic nervous system. Several studies have demonstrated that hypnosis helps regulate autonomic balance, often by activating the parasympathetic branch, the one that calms us down. It may also downregulate the sympathetic system—the activating branch that carries out the fight–flight response. This combination can be very helpful for reducing autonomic dysregulation. Occasionally, hypnosis helps by up–regulating the sympathetic branch.

One important study (Dillworth, Mendoza, and Jensen, 2012) suggests that hypnosis is able to disrupt pain because it alters the brain's pain network. (Refer back to Chapter 2, "How Pain Works in Your Brain and Nervous System," for a discussion of the pain network.)

It seems to be that activating these brain regions through hypnosis allows for some of the beneficial changes that we see in our patients. For example, hypnosis may allow for the ability to focus deeply on hypnotic suggestions without distraction, and the ability to experience actual physical changes through a hypnotic suggestion.

Some research has monitored brain wave activity during hypnosis. Several studies have shown a high frequency of theta waves, which are often observed during deep relaxation, daydreaming, or focused concentration. This supports the idea that hypnosis is different than a sleep state. These studies also suggest that people who are more susceptible to hypnosis show greater theta activity than those who are not susceptible.

So what does all that mean? As a practitioner, this research suggests that different sorts of hypnotic suggestions can tap into different areas of the brain. It all depends on the purpose of the suggestion: reducing the intensity of pain, decreasing anxiety or depression associated with pain, improving sleep quality, spurring interest in physical activity, and so on.

Part of what makes hypnosis such a valuable treatment for chronic pain is that it can affect multiple pain-related outcomes. Hypnosis can decrease pain, increase comfort, improve the ability to ignore pain, or shift attention away from pain. One can even learn to change the sensation of pain to another sensation, such as tingling or numbness. More broadly, suggestions may focus on improvements in other areas of life that affect the experience of pain—or vice versa. Suggestions can be used to improve self-confidence, to become more involved in activities of daily living, to change beliefs or attitudes, or to improve self-care habits.

Even though hypnosis can provide comfort and relief for the chronic pain sufferer, it doesn't mean that the pain was psychosomatic or all in your head. Hypnosis works through its effects on multiple pathways through the brain and nervous system.

WHAT HAPPENS IN THE HYPNOTIC EXPERIENCE

Since clinical hypnosis is not a standalone therapy, the decision to use it is made in the overall context of the patient's therapeutic program and objectives. Perhaps the most important aspect of entering the hypnotic experience is the quality of the therapeutic relationship between doctor and patient. The first step in the process of using hypnosis is a thorough discussion between the two to clarify the patient's goals for healing from chronic pain. Your answers to the pain assessment will guide how we work together with hypnosis.

THE THREE STAGES OF HYPNOSIS

There are many variables that make each session of clinical hypnosis unique, but they typically follow the same basic three-stage structure: induction, application, and the re-alerting phase.

Induction Phase

Hypnosis begins with the *induction* phase. In the movies, this is where the hypnotist swings a pocket watch back and forth or uses some other device to focus the attention of the subject. Medically trained hypnotist-clinicians seldom use such clichés to guide the subject into a calm and receptive state of mind. I have adopted the common practice of having you focus on your breath as a way to begin the experience. Another common option is to have you stare at a fixed object in the room. The type of induction used varies depending on the individual patient and type of problem. During induction, you focus your attention away from any thoughts or abstractions and gradually fall into a trance state.

Application Phase

The *application* phase comes once you have achieved a receptive state of mind. I will address the goals you have selected for treatment by making various suggestions. Your goal may be, "reduce my headache intensity," "sleep through the night better," or "feel less trapped by the pain and more hopeful." We may address several goals. One of the wonderful things about hypnosis is that one hypnotic session can include suggestions for many therapeutic objectives—such as decreased pain, increased comfort, improved sleep, improved interest in practicing self-care exercises, etc.

Some of my suggestions are direct, such as "You will have reduced pain and increased comfort in your neck." Other times I will use metaphorical suggestions that are more indirect. I may say, "Notice how the dark storm clouds start to diminish, revealing a beautiful blue sky underneath."

Another powerful strategy in clinical hypnosis is the use of *post-hypnotic suggestions*. This is a helpful tool to incline you toward desired changes in the future. An example of a post-hypnotic suggestion would be, "And every time that you listen to this recording, you will find even more relaxation and comfort and will look forward to practicing this even more regularly." When we use hypnosis for treating chronic pain, post-hypnotic suggestions often have you "picture yourself in the future with more comfort and flexibility, being able to return to more and more desired activities of daily living."

We typically record your hypnosis session so you can practice it at home every day. That way it becomes an ongoing part of your healing process. The only time I don't record the session is when the purpose of the hypnosis is exploratory. On rare occasions, patients sometimes decide it would be beneficial for me to probe into some of their deeper feelings or concerns regarding the pain, or to explore unforeseen barriers to their progress. I use exploratory hypnosis only with your consent and only after a frank and open discussion about whether it would be useful.

Re-Alerting Phase

The last step in the hypnosis progress is the *re-alerting* phase. I facilitate a smooth, gentle transition from the hypnotic trance to normal wakefulness. This phase may last from thirty seconds to several minutes. Many patients tell me that the hypnotic state was so comfortable that they'd rather stay in it much longer! Once you are back in a wakeful state, we discuss your experience. You can tell me what the hypnosis was like for you, ask questions, and possibly have new insights about your pain and healing.

SUSAN'S FIRST HYPNOSIS EXPERIENCE

Susan was a relatively new patient, but we had come to a point in her treatment where hypnosis seemed like a good next step. She was a fifty-three-year-old business executive with chronic pain who had spent ten years seeing numerous physicians, chiropractors, and massage therapists.

Several years ago she had surgery to correct a herniated disc, but that didn't stop the pain. She described it as an ongoing, low-grade deep ache across her entire low back, with occasional spikes of sharp stabbing pain in her buttocks and hips. Every so often she'd have a burning sciatic pain radiate down her left leg. By the time she came to me, Susan felt like she had run out of options and was ready to try something new.

When I first told her about hypnosis, she was open to the idea, but was rather dubious.

"I'm quite sure I'm not hypnotizable," Susan said. "I do best when I maintain full control, and I can't imagine letting go of that."

"That might be true," I told her. "But let's proceed and just see what happens."

People do vary in their ability to be hypnotized. If you really resist the idea, then you won't fall into a trance. But people are not always the best judge of whether they are hypnotizable or not. I think the major factor is whether they are willing. We have a saying in the hypnosis field: "All hypnosis is self-hypnosis."

What follows is an abbreviated version of Susan's first hypnosis experience. The typical session lasts for about twenty minutes.

I dimmed the lights and had Susan sit comfortably in an easy chair. I spoke to her in a gentle, reassuring manner.

"Start with your eyes open and take a few deep breaths···"

I paused for about half a minute to let her develop her rhythm of deep breaths. Frequent pauses—anywhere from five seconds to a minute or more—are an important ingredient in the procedure. They slow the pace and give the subject ample time to focus on their feelings and sensations.

"Eventually you may find it more comfortable for your eyes to stay comfortably closed··· Good··· No effort required, nothing you need to do··· Just notice as the relaxation and comfort spread easily with every breath···"

Contrary to her suspicions, Susan was becoming quite relaxed.

"And now, if you'd like to experience an even deeper level of comfort and healing, we are going to count down from ten to one···"

By the time I reached one, Susan had reached a receptive hypnotic state. She was pleasantly surprised to find this sense of calm, even though she did not feel "out of it." She still knew who she was and where she was.

She felt a deepening sense of calm throughout her chest, abdomen, and legs. Her arms and hands were feeling increasingly heavy and warm, and a little tingly. She could still hear my voice, but it was drifting more and more into the background.

Then I engaged her imagination with a visualization.

"And now···if you'd like to experience yet an even deeper level of relaxation, relief, and comfort···I'm going to invite you to picture that you are sunbathing in one of your favorite places··· You can feel the gentle warmth of the sun soothe and comfort your low back···"

Susan found herself relaxing on the dock of her summer cabin on a pleasant summer day. But she thought to herself, "There's no way that my back is going to feel any differently."

"Whatever scene you see right now, see it in close, vivid detail, as if you are actually there right now··· Allow yourself to fully let in the beauty surrounding you."

Despite her skepticism, Susan's body and emotions were responding to the hypnotic suggestions.

"And now···without any effort at all···allow a gentle wave of relaxation···just like a gentle wave or ripple on a lake···to bring an increasing sense of comfort···calming···balance···healing···relaxation···"

To her surprise, Susan felt the tension unwinding in her low back. The deep ache faded for the first time in months!

While she was still in the trance, I gave her a post-hypnotic suggestion.

"Isn't it good to know···that a deeper part of you···is learning this sense of healing···deep comfort···and relaxation?··· It can help you return to this state more effectively···every time that you practice this···and a deeper part of you···can sense exactly where the relief is needed most···"

Eventually it was time to bring her back to her normal state of alertness.

"We are going to count again, and this time, from one to ten··· And when we reach ten, you can bring your attention totally back to *this* room where you are sitting now···feeling relaxed and refreshed and feeling good about your experience···"

After she opened her eyes and her mind was back in my office, we started discussing her experience.

"How long did you think it lasted?" I asked.

"Oh, about eight or ten minutes," she replied.

"Well, if you look at the clock you can see that twenty minutes went by." She looked at the clock in disbelief and we both started laughing.

"Tell me about your experience."

"A part of me was able to stand back and observe the whole thing—what you were saying, even what I thought about what you were saying. But meanwhile, I noticed very interesting changes occurring internally."

We continued our talk for a while and then I gave her a recording of the session for her to use at home. She made a practice of listening to it every day. After a month or so she told me, "My back pain hasn't entirely disappeared, but the hypnosis has really turned down the intensity so that I can get back to more of my daily activities!"

CHAPTER 24

Resolving Difficult Emotions and Their Physical Effects

MEDICINE'S PROGRESS IN HEALING THE MIND-BODY SPLIT

"Is my chronic pain real or psychosomatic?"

The world of modern medicine has traditionally considered only two categories of symptoms. Only one type was thought to be real. Real symptoms are the physical ones you can verify by examining the body or running a test. These organic physical symptoms can be measured, quantified, and traced back to some bodily condition.

But if the reported symptoms do not show up on tests, or if they are out of proportion to the test results, then they must not be real. They aren't caused by your body, so they must come from your mind. Such so-called psychological symptoms are often referred to as stress-related or psychosomatic symptoms. The connotations of these words haunt patients who report such symptoms. These words seem to blame them for a problem they didn't cause. Because it's "all in their head."

Our natural healing capacities can bring clarity and restoration to these syndromes referred to as so-called *psychosomatic illnesses*. The common denominator of these disorders is that they are said to be caused strictly by unresolved emotional conflicts. I agree that emotional conflicts may play a contributing role, but they are not a sufficient cause by themselves. Rather, most often it starts with a physical vulnerability that is then worsened by emotional conflicts.

I have already mentioned that categorizing symptoms as psychosomatic is misleading, but it is part of a tradition that began four hundred years ago. Viewing illness with a sharp distinction between real physical symptoms and unreal psychological symptoms dates back to Descartes. He's the French philosopher whose mechanistic theory of pain guided modern medicine's treatment of pain until the 1960s. Descartes famously promoted the idea that the mind and the body are completely separate entities.

Descartes's mind–body split suited the scientists in the emerging fields of medicine and physiology. They focused only on the body and its diseases. The mind had nothing to do with it. They were content to let others deal with the mind: philosophers, theologians, and eventually, psychologists and psychiatrists. Descartes drew a sharp line between the body and mind, and that line persists in the traditional medical paradigm. It is only now being changed.

In recent decades we have discovered that the mind connects with the body at the cellular level. Each emotion that we experience is born as an electrical nerve and hormone signal. Depending on the type of emotion, the nerve signals produce various chemical hormones made from protein. They are called neuropeptides. These chemicals are secreted into the bloodstream, where they serve as messenger molecules. They deliver their message to every cell in the body. Depending on the emotion, certain cells react to it—giving you a physiological response. This sequence explains how what goes on in the mind has a physical impact on the body.

Difficult or stressful emotions give rise to neuropeptides that can weaken your body's immune system. That is why we are more likely to catch a cold or other infection during or directly after an emotionally difficult time. So when we feel upset, anxious, or stressed, our health can suffer. Today we know how thoughts and emotions concretely interact with behavior and physiology. There is no line between them.

The discovery of the mind–body connection was the culmination of a series of scientific breakthroughs throughout the twentieth century. These seminal discoveries—clustered around the immune system and nervous system—have revolutionized our understanding of mind–body connections: Dr. Hans Selye proving that stress plays an important role in physical illness. Dr. George Engel demonstrating that health and illness result from a combination of biological, psychological, and social factors. Dr. Robert Ader's contribution that the immune system is influenced by the autonomic nervous system, and that the immune system can actually *learn*.

Dr. Ader's research created the field known as *psychoneuroimmunology*: the study of how the mind and the stress response affect the ability of the immune system to maintain health and fight disease. We now know that emotions and behavioral reactions can influence physical illness or health through communication with the nervous system, hormonal system, and immune system. Science has evolved to demonstrate that emotions and thoughts can cause physiological changes in the body.

The traditional biomedical model excludes emotions and feelings as irrelevant in understanding "real" symptoms. That's why it is so common for providers and patients alike to misunderstand the important interactions between emotions and chronic pain. Nevertheless, chronic pain sufferers are often told that their problem is an emotional one. Until you connect the dots of what this means, there is often defensiveness about the role of feelings. Patients are apt to say, "If you talk about my emotions, then you are implying that my chronic pain is all in my head and not real!"

And yet it is well–known that chronic pain affects your emotions, and your emotions affect your pain. Negative emotions add to your suffering when pain makes you angry, sad, anxious or stressed. Positive emotions, however, can have a beneficial effect. Sometimes you forget all about the pain in your back when you are engaged in doing fun things—such as attending a live concert, or playing with your grandchildren. When you are enjoying yourself and feeling happy, you hardly notice your pain. The ways that your mind modulates thoughts and emotions affect the ways that your body controls pain.

To add to your suffering, pain and the fear of pain can cause you to avoid physical and social activities that you normally enjoy. This sort of reclusive withdrawal can weaken your relationships, reduce your mobility, and then contribute to the vicious cycle of more chronic pain. Pain can cause depression and anxiety, and conversely the presence of depression or anxiety can make your existing pain worse. The result is that depression and anxiety are very common among people living with chronic pain.

The connection between chronic pain and difficult emotions is not just a coincidence. From a neurological perspective, we can see that both emotions and pain are processed by the same structures in the brain. The areas of our brain that are associated with sensory pain perception overlap with the areas of the brain that process emotions. That means in order to heal from chronic pain, we must first understand what happens in the normal functioning of emotions. And then we must face the challenge of processing difficult emotions.

Emotions are a naturally occurring phenomenon in all mammals. We are hardwired to experience emotions, both positive ones and negative ones. Positive emotions include excitement, happiness, and tenderness, while negative emotions refer to such feelings as sadness, anger, and fear. Emotions each have their own life cycle. When you can allow yourself to experience the feeling in your body, the emotion is eventually discharged, and you can move on. You've gotten over it. However, when you can't or won't allow yourself to experience the emotion, it often becomes stuck. There are lots of reasons why we sometimes resist experiencing feelings of sadness or anxiety. Perhaps we avoid them because they make us feel uncomfortable. Maybe we instinctively fear that the emotion will weaken us, or that we will sink into a bottomless well of grief.

One thing is for sure. When you fight the feeling, problems ensue. For example, when you chronically fight or deny the experience of anger or sadness in your body, it may eventually manifest in the form of depression.

There is no better illustration of this than looking at an infant. One moment the baby is angry and screaming, and then before you know it she is laughing with delight. They don't hold anything back. They fully express each bout of sadness and happiness. But we almost never see a depressed infant! This is because the infant has not yet learned to suppress feelings of anger or sadness. That allows the ongoing flow of whatever feeling surfaces! Babies possess the natural ability to go with the flow of their emotions. Somehow, we learn to fight that natural ability as we grow older.

What happens to us physically when we don't effectively process our emotions? One of the best lessons I have learned on this topic comes from a presentation by Dr. Robert Scaer, a neurologist who studies the effects of post-traumatic stress. At a conference where we were teaching together, Dr. Scaer showed a video that powerfully conveys the effects of trauma on behavior in the animal kingdom. He began his program with a question. Why don't wild animals exhibit the symptoms of PTSD? After all, their lives are filled with life-threatening trauma—they struggle to survive as both predator and prey.

His video was a documentary on researchers in the Arctic who were investigating the effects of a traumatic stimulus on polar bears. The scientists aboard a helicopter sighted a group of polar bears. The noise of the helicopter frightened them, and they ran away. They flew low enough to shoot one of the fleeing bears with a tranquilizer dart. They landed and approached the tranquilized polar bear, who lay motionless on the ground. Later, after they had conducted their examination, the tranquilizer gradually wore off. The bear opened his eyes and became alert, but remained motionless. Dr. Scaer likens this to a post-traumatic "freeze response." A short time later, the bear started trembling uncontrollably. The shaking lasted for nearly an hour. All of a sudden, the bear got up on all four legs and walked away as if nothing had ever happened!

Scaer interprets this bizarre scene as depicting a crucial distinction between humans and wild animals. Animals in the wild have never learned to hide or suppress negative emotions or physiological reactions such as the uncontrollable trembling. The frenzied shaking is a way to discharge the nervous system, releasing the psychophysiological effects of trauma.

It is one of the great contradictions of civilized human culture that we have learned to suppress our emotional reactions even though it is bad for our health. It is simply not socially acceptable to go around crying or trembling with fear. What would people think? As a result, our nervous systems don't have the opportunity to discharge the trauma. That leads to unresolved tension, nightmares, and feelings of dread that accompany both PTSD and chronic anxiety. I tell my patients this story to show the importance of allowing physical expressions of emotions when they arise— whether it's crying, blushing, or even trembling with anxiety. I tell them that crying is just as important a nervous system discharge as trembling is for that polar bear!

WHAT HAPPENS PHYSICALLY WHEN WE SUPPRESS AN EMOTION?

Let's imagine once again that you are in a social situation where you want to hide your emotions. Although you are on the verge of tears, you must attend a social function at work. As you enter the room where your coworkers have gathered, you don't want them to know that you feel like crying. How would you guard against that? The customary strategy is to "grit your teeth and bear it" or "keep a stiff upper lip." Physically speaking, donning a facial mask to hide your feelings is a matter of tightening your muscles of expression—e.g. the muscles and tissues of your face, neck, and upper chest. You would want to tighten the muscles around your jaw and mouth, so others don't see your lips trembling. To avoid crying, you'd tighten the muscles around your eyes, temples, and forehead. Your breathing would shift to shallow upper chest breaths, since we instinctively know that deep belly breaths are more likely to bring those deeper emotions up to the surface.

But what if you must keep up this ruse for a long time? When you chronically control the expression of difficult emotions, you have to keep all those muscles in a constant state of tense readiness. Each morning you brace yourself for another exhausting day of tight muscles and restricted breathing. Imagine how, over time, this could contribute to continued symptoms of chronic pain and fatigue.

Suppressing your emotions is a double-edged sword. When you successfully block out your negative emotions, it also keeps the positive feelings from coming through. I saw a good example of this in a patient who had chronic arm pain. In response to the pain, she developed chronic depression and hopelessness. The stronger her pain, the more hopelessness she felt. Over time she learned to suppress that emotional response. She hated feeling helpless, so she denied her feelings to the point where she became emotionally dulled. But then she couldn't feel any emotion—good or bad. Because of this, whenever she encountered any improvement, she was unable to feel good about it. She had no sense of hope, relief, or encouragement, and these feelings are necessary to cope with the ongoing rehabilitation from chronic pain. She had developed what I call "prudent pessimism." Or, as the lyric from the rock song goes, "Things don't seem as dark when you're already dressed in black."

When it comes to the somber duet of emotional problems and chronic pain, it does not matter which comes first. Sometimes emotional problems predate the onset of chronic pain. A person could suffer from chronic depression for years and then develop chronic migraine headaches. Or someone could get injured at work and go on Workers' Compensation for years with low back pain, only to develop chronic irritability and anxiety after being confined to his home for several months. Whether the chronic pain or the emotional difficulties developed first doesn't really matter. Both are normal, common reactions.

THE HEALING POWER OF TEARS

The list of unpleasant emotions one can experience from chronic pain is long indeed. They include anger, frustration, inadequacy, fear, guilt, shame, anxiety, and overwhelm, to name just a few.

And yet, the most difficult emotion for most people that I have seen over the years is sadness. This feeling, along with its variants—grief, loss, emptiness—seem to be the one that causes the biggest problems and generates the most resistance.

There are many reasons for this. Anger and anxiety are *activating* emotions. These feelings are associated with arousal, elevated heart rate, and muscle tension. These emotions help mobilize the fight–flight response in the body. They are part of our innate trauma response that prepares us to do battle or to escape as quickly as possible. By contrast, sadness and loss are associated with the opposite response—a deep sense of emptiness, grief, isolation, and weakness. Rather than stimulating a mobilization response, sadness and loss often feel as if the bottom has dropped out. Sadness, therefore, can feel far more vulnerable than other emotions.

Psychodynamic theorists have written about this phenomenon for years. Alexander Lowen, a psychiatrist, developed the field of analysis known as bioenergetics. This approach asserted that emotional problems arose from chronic muscular bracing and guarding in the body due to excessive stress. Understanding the mind–body connection was central to his approach, and his treatment focused on how difficult emotions are stored in the body.

In particular, Lowen stressed that we grow up being taught to inhibit crying, because it conveys weakness, or immaturity. As someone learns to guard against crying, they also learn to guard against the letting–go that happens with experiencing pleasure. In effect, we learn to hold ourselves rigidly, including tight, rigid muscles. Lowen said that we maintain this physical rigidity as a way to block out painful sensations as well as painful emotions.

In our culture, children are commonly taught to restrain their emotions. Above all, they are not supposed to cry. Many children can remember being teased in elementary school for crying when they got hurt. Some parents threaten their children with the admonition, "Stop crying or I'll give you something to cry about." Many people grow up believing that crying is a sign of weakness. Such tearful behavior also places a burden on people close to them. The phrase "boys don't cry" is widely understood and was even the title of a major motion picture. The prohibition against crying, however, is widely upheld by both sexes.

Paradoxically, even though crying is often discouraged in our culture, the value of a good cry for feeling better is widely understood. The significance of releasing deeply stored grief and loss has been recognized not only in psychological circles, but in pop culture as well. You might remember the chart-topping group Tears For Fears and their number-one hit single "Everybody Wants to Rule the World." The co-leaders of the group explained in interviews that they chose their name based on their experiences in psychotherapy. They learned that by accepting their anxiety instead of fighting it, they could let go and cry to resolve their underlying sadness. By accepting their tears, they reduced their fears.

CHRONIC PAIN, SADNESS, AND LOSS

The sense of loss is obvious after the death of a loved one, but that feeling of loss is also common with chronic pain. The fear of being incapacitated by pain can feel like the fear of death itself. Patients with chronic pain experience profound losses because of the multiple impacts it has on their lives. After all, chronic pain can cause a loss of abilities and roles, job-related losses, and financial losses. One can even suffer a loss of identity—feeling changed as a person and misunderstood by others.

WHY DO WE CRY?

Crying emotional tears has the potential of multiple health benefits. We are not speaking of reflex tears, which occur when you get something in your eye, or the continuous tears that keep your eyes lubricated. Emotional tears are released at times of strong emotion, particularly sadness or joy. These tears help self-soothing, but they are also important for biological homeostasis. Such tears prompt the release of beneficial neurohormones such as oxytocin, serotonin (mood-enhancing), and endorphins (natural painkillers). Crying emotional tears also helps balance the activating and calming branches of our autonomic nervous system. Research has revealed that crying may also serve more complex communication and social bonding functions.

RELEASE AND BALANCE: THE EMOTIONAL AND PHYSIOLOGICAL VALUE OF CRYING

Crying is a hardwired automatic process for self-regulation and biological homeostasis.

We are all born with the capacity to experience a wide variety of emotional states. These include positive emotions such as happiness, excitement, and joy, and negative emotions such as sadness, anger, and fear. As I mentioned earlier, when you notice an emotion surface and allow it to be there without struggle, the feeling eventually passes.

Consider sadness—a normal response to grief or loss. When we let the feelings and sensations of sadness be experienced without avoidance or struggle, eventually the sadness passes. But if you were to chronically suppress feelings of sadness, it would eventually morph into clinical depression. Instead of a transitory sadness, you become immersed in a constellation of despair, exhaustion, insomnia, appetite disturbance, and hopelessness. That is often treated with psychotherapy and antidepressant medication.

Just as Dr. Scaer's polar bear taught us, physical expression of difficult emotions allows for nervous system regulation. Such a release is essential for healing from the trauma of chronic pain.

Irene is a ninety-year-old woman who has been suffering from chronic low back pain for several years. She is very bright intellectually, but has had difficulty identifying anything more than the most basic emotions, with anxiety being the most common one she suffered from. In the course of her treatment with me, she worked diligently to pay more attention to the sensations and emotions of her body, making significant progress. As our work together progressed, she became more aware of feelings of deep grief and loss about all she has missed out on because of being so limited due to back pain.

I introduced the concept of the healing power of tears to Irene. At first, she was skeptical about this. "Of course I know I'm sad about this—what good will it do to cry over spilled milk?" She reluctantly agreed to do this exercise with me. I encouraged her to start with a brief 4-4-8 breathing technique. Then I guided her to take slow, steady breaths as she let herself acknowledge all that she has missed out on due to her back pain. After a minute or so, her lower lip started to quiver, and soon she was crying. I encouraged her not to have to "understand why" and instead just allow this natural bodily reaction to occur. This went on for about one or two minutes. The crying naturally ended. Then what followed was very surprising to Irene. She said: "I never would have believed it—my anxiety is gone, and the back pain is less than half of what it was when I began the exercise!"

Months later, my check-in with Irene revealed that her daily practice of allowing tears is paying big dividends. "I allow myself to have tears every morning for just a few minutes. I can feel how much calmer my mind and body feel afterwards. If I happen to miss a day of practice, I notice because my back pain gets ornery again! I hope you are teaching this to all of your patients!"

HOW TO REGAIN THE CAPACITY
TO SHED EMOTIONAL TEARS

Now that you know the health benefits of crying, how can you allow yourself to do it, especially if you are not used to allowing tears?

Happily, there are several strategies available to regain this inborn ability.

Start by taking a short walk—even three to five minutes walking will help by releasing some of the chronic muscular guarding that prevents crying. Follow this with one of the following strategies:

• Listen to emotionally evocative music.

- Watch movies that have made you cry in the past. If you need more choices, do a Google search for "the best sad movies." One recent online search revealed "Seventy-Seven Best Sad Movies to Cry To."

- Think of your saddest memories: the death of a loved one, or a time when you felt hurt by someone close to you. You may feel hesitant to do this, but the resulting release will make you feel better.

- Think about what you are grateful for.

DO EMOTIONS OCCUR IN YOUR HEAD—OR IN YOUR BODY?

People often talk as if emotions occur in their head, as if they are some sort of mental activity. A physician who can't find a physical cause for your symptoms might say, "It's all in your head." A derogatory way to refer to someone with emotional problems is to call them a "head case." People accused of being emotionally unstable may hear, "You ought to have your head examined!"

Aside from being offensive, these expressions are not grounded in scientific fact. The truth is that the only place that you can experience emotion is in your body. That holds for any emotional experience you can imagine. Emotions may be triggered in your brain, but they are not felt in your brain.

When an emotion happens, the brain sends a series of messenger molecules throughout your body. The chemical composition of these molecules varies depending on the emotion, but each message contains a program that causes physiological changes that ready us for action. We can sense these changes physically by paying attention to our bodies. For example, you know you're in love from the warm feeling in your heart, and the smile that just won't quit. You know you're anxious by feeling your heart racing, your mouth becoming dry, your skin turning pale, and your muscles contracting. When you feel sad, your body feels heavy, or you can sense an aching emptiness in your chest. Feeling emotions is a matter of reading the body.

An interesting example of this misconception about emotions involves the neurotransmitter *serotonin*. It is a widely known mood–enhancer that improves the experiences of depression and anxiety. Some antidepressant medications work in part by adjusting the amount of serotonin between nerves. Many people naturally think that most receptors for serotonin are in the brain. Perhaps it will surprise you to know that over 95 percent of all serotonin receptors are located in the gut! This is just one of many examples of how emotions are intertwined with the body.

A jumble of difficult emotions can become associated with chronic pain. Some feel deep sadness and grief at their sorry state. A strong desire for relief may cause feelings of intense anxiety and impatience. You might feel angry and resentful when you see everyone happily going about their day, oblivious to your burden of chronic pain. It might be feelings of shame and embarrassment. Some feel jealous toward all the others who doesn't have to struggle so much.

Regardless of which emotion becomes commingled with your chronic pain, the result is greater suffering. Think of the physical changes in your body if you had a deep, aching chronic pain in your lower back. You may get occasional tingling or burning down one leg. Just the effort of cautiously moving your sore body around all day leaves your muscles feeling stiff and tired. Add the physical manifestations of sadness, anxiety, and frustration that are so common with chronic pain. The net effect is often an experience of *overwhelm* and *despair*.

Knowing how to work effectively with these difficult emotions can ease the intensity of suffering in chronic pain. The place to begin is by understanding that your emotions are *embodied*.

Now that you know something about how difficult emotions can negatively affect chronic pain, we will explore what recent research tells us about how past emotional difficulties can affect your pain.

ADVERSE CHILDHOOD EXPERIENCES AND CHRONIC PAIN

Some of my new patients are a bit puzzled when I ask them whether they had experienced any sort of childhood trauma. They wonder to themselves, "What in the world does childhood trauma have to do with my chronic pain problem?" It can have a lot to do with it. Many studies indicate that someone who has experienced adverse childhood experiences (ACEs) are two to three times more likely to develop chronic pain as an adult. That's why I ask about their childhoods. It can be a significant factor in chronic pain, and it affects a lot of people. Once we know about such things, however, we can address them in treatment.

THE PSYCHOLOGICAL AND PHYSIOLOGICAL EFFECTS OF ADVERSE CHILDHOOD EXPERIENCES (ACES)

The idea that childhood trauma can have long-lasting psychological effects is as old as Freud. The updated version is that ACEs can have physiological effects as well.

In 1997, the Centers for Disease Control (CDC) teamed up with healthcare conglomerate Kaiser Permanente for a groundbreaking study of the effects of childhood abuse, neglect, and dysfunctional homes. They sorted these various problems into a list of ten adverse childhood experiences, or ACEs. They were looking for things that affected a child anywhere from birth to their eighteenth birthday.

They found that ACEs are quite common. About 61 percent of adults surveyed across twenty-five states reported experiencing at least one type of ACE and nearly 17 percent reported that they had at least four ACEs. The CDC–Kaiser Permanente study found that ACEs create a major negative impact on general mental and physical health conditions in adulthood. Resulting maladies such as heart disease and depression have enormous social and economic costs for families, communities, and society.

Examples of ACEs include:

- Witnessing violence in the home or community

- Experiencing violence, abuse, or emotional neglect

- Having a family member attempt or die by suicide

- Growing up in a problematic home with

  - Substance abuse

  - Mental health problems

  - Parental separation or divorce

  - Household members in jail or prison

HOW DO ACES CONTRIBUTE TO CHRONIC PAIN?

ACEs create a complex mix of psychological changes and physiological changes in the brain and nervous system that add to the risk of developing or worsening chronic pain. These changes fit within our previous discussion of stress, and how too much stress can damage the function of our central stress-response system, the HPA axis.

When someone experiences *chronic* traumatic events such as ACEs, the HPA system may be chronically activated and dysregulated, leading to increased wear and tear on the body and mind. Over time, this dysregulation can negatively affect learning, behavior, and emotional regulation—all of which can lead to heightened vulnerability to developing chronic pain.

Over time, ACEs can affect parts of the brain that we refer to as the pain network. This can cause parts of our limbic brain to become overly sensitive to threats. Our alarm system can be set off by a stimulus that is ordinarily too weak to evoke a response. At the same time, ACEs can weaken the ability of your rational brain (frontal cortex) to calm down the faulty alarm. The systemic weakening of these brain functions can lead to problems later in life—inflammation in the body, increased pain sensitivity, and greater severity of pain.

In addition to having these physical effects on the brain, ACEs also have psychological consequences. These can also contribute to chronic pain. ACEs can lead to catastrophizing, feeling powerless, feeling generally unwell physically, and feeling lonely. More broadly, ACEs are linked to a greater prevalence of depression and anxiety. People with those conditions are twice as likely to develop chronic pain.

WHAT CAN BE DONE FOR THE CHRONIC PAIN SUFFERER WITH A HISTORY OF ACES?

There are many ways to heal both the psychological and neurophysiological changes that result from ACEs. Many of the treatment strategies for ACEs overlap with our other tools for addressing chronic pain, the ABC method.

The general goal for those with a history of ACEs is to increase resilience, the ability to cope with the ongoing daily stresses of life. Greater resilience can be achieved by improving physical, emotional, and social health. This requires developing problem-solving skills and self-regulation abilities.

Here is a list of treatment areas to keep in mind:

- **Bodily self-care:** Obtaining appropriate sleep, nutrition, exercise

- **Emotional self-care:** Developing coping skills for dealing with difficult emotions:

  - Identifying when you are numb

  - Overcoming sensory dissociation

  - Nurturing self-compassion—so that you feel entitled to self-care

  - Practicing self-soothing and self-regulation skills

- **Cognitive self-care:** Recognizing and reflecting on problematic beliefs—especially those that are self-limiting, self-critical, and self-sabotaging

- **Socialization:** Developing interpersonal skills that foster productive relationships, including communication skills and setting boundaries

Here are some useful tools for improving self-care:

- **Journal writing:** A way to identify and deal with negative emotions

- **Mindfulness meditation:** Promotes generalized calming, aids emotional regulation, enables "big picture" perspective

- **Clinical hypnosis:** Improves mood and cognitive clarity, reduces hypervigilance and impulsivity, increases capacity for self-soothing and self-regulation

WHAT TO DO ABOUT NEGATIVE EMOTIONS

Now that you know the importance of dealing with negative emotions for your chronic pain, what do you do about it? There are a lot of myths and misconceptions about this. A common misconception is the "pressure cooker" metaphor. According to this model, your suppressed feelings build up more and more pressure until they finally explode—in the form of a tantrum or emotional breakdown. The only way to prevent such a blowout is to release the pressure or blow off some steam by yelling, screaming, beating on a pillow, or confronting someone head-on. The pressure-cooker model is ineffective because it doesn't accurately depict how emotions work.

As I wrote in my earlier book, *Trust Your Gut*, the way to resolve the effects of negative emotions is to call on the power of your self-awareness skills. The key is to first recognize negative feelings, and then express them.

These two steps sound surprisingly simple, but are very effective when applied regularly:

TWO-STEP SYSTEM FOR RESOLVING NEGATIVE EMOTIONS

1. **Recognize:** Acknowledge the emotion to yourself and feel it physically in your body

2. **Express:** Choose from a wide continuum of possible constructive actions to resolve the suppressed emotion

Let's take a closer look at each of these steps.

STEP ONE: RECOGNIZE

Recognizing an emotion means identifying the feeling in your body and acknowledging to yourself that the feeling is there. It may be a suppressed emotion or an unmet need from the past. If you continue to ignore it, it may become a major trigger for future pain flare-ups. But when you allow yourself to feel these difficult emotions, then you can resolve them and promote healing. Recognizing the emotion is the first step in this process.

How do you do this? Start by asking this question: "What do I feel?" It may take a while for the answer to emerge, so be patient and allow some time for it to come to awareness. Observe the thoughts that pop up as well as the sensations that you notice in your body. Don't judge—just watch, listen, and feel.

Don't Ask Why

When you are trying to recognize a difficult emotion, do not ask why the feeling is there. Asking that question activates different parts of the brain than the ones you are using to recognize the feeling. As you stay with the experience without judging, the reasons why the feeling is there will soon become clearer.

Methods to Help Recognize Your Emotions

Emotions are important because they are reliable indicators of your inner state. The goal is to find methods for recognizing your emotions that best fit your personality. Some people need to be around trusted others to get in touch with this, while others do better through solitude.

These strategies will help you recognize what you are feeling:

- **Limbic Retraining:** The same powerful method for reducing the distress of chronic pain also works very well for recognizing your emotions. The first step is to stop and recognize that you may be feeling something. It may start as a hunch or inkling that something is stirred up. Once you recognize a little feeling of sadness, anxiety, or anger, then scan your body and notice where you can tangibly sense the feeling. Using Limbic Retraining is a good reminder that feeling refers to both emotion and bodily sensations. Find the part of your body where you most notice the trace of this feeling, whether a rumbling in your abdomen or a tightness in your arms or chest. Focus on the sensation without trying to change it. Stay with it as it moves and changes. Refer to the section on Limbic Retraining in this book (Chapter 22) for more tips on using this method.

- **Pay attention to your thoughts and daydreams.** This will reveal a lot to you about your life, your relationships, your loves and hates. Write down these snippets of daydreams and thoughts because writing them down will bring a greater level of awareness of patterns and clues about your emotional experience.

- **Identify the minor hurts that may seem little and unimportant.** Many people routinely brush off these hurts, saying, "It doesn't matter" or, "It's not important." That's a mistake, because big pieces of hurt emotion are buried within them, so these minor hurts do matter. Men in particular are socialized to frequently downplay what bothers them. These buried emotions can create difficulties with your health by triggering imbalances in your nervous system that can worsen your pain. Identifying these hurts will reveal much to you about unrecognized difficult feelings.

- **Write in a journal.** Keep an ongoing record of any noticeable emotions. (Refer to the section in this book on journal writing in Chapter 11). Research tells us that briefly writing down the emotion—without regard to *why* you are feeling it—can make you feel better and reduce a potential pain trigger.

- **Notice memories that recur and don't go away.** If you repeatedly remember situations or hurts that happened long ago, you are guaranteed to have unresolved emotions toward the person or situation. Document these awarenesses carefully as they are likely contributing to increased physical pain.

- **Be specific:** As you learn to recognize your emotions, you might get stuck by using terms that are too general. For example, consider depression. What you are calling depression may be more accurately described as sadness, loneliness, boredom, a lack of creativity in your life, abandonment, or suppressed anger. The more specifically you can identify and label your feeling, the easier it will be to resolve it.

- **Be aware of excessive or compulsive behaviors.** This is especially important if this pattern has emerged in recent weeks or months. Overeating, overworking, drinking daily, or compulsive sex or gambling are examples. You may be acting this way because you are avoiding unpleasant feelings that emerge when you stop the behavior. Noticing this can help in recognizing the underlying feeling.

- **Expand your emotional vocabulary.** Examples of feeling words include angry, sad, scared, happy, excited, tender, ashamed, amused, terrified, impatient, rageful, giddy, appreciative, grateful, calm, agitated, joyful, weary. This is not, of course, an all-inclusive list, but may serve as a useful starting point for identifying your emotional experience. To exercise your "emotion muscles," start a daily practice of writing briefly in a journal on "What am I feeling right now?" With practice, you will more readily find terms that fit your experience.

- **Notice your positive emotions.** These may include love, compassion, excitement, tenderness, and joy. The way that our emotions are hardwired, you cannot suppress just one emotion without suppressing all of them. By recognizing the positive emotions that you experience, you will help to open the pathways to recognizing negative emotions as well.

STEP TWO: EXPRESS

Once you have recognized the emotion you are feeling, the next step is to decide what type of action (if any) is needed to express the emotion. Resolving negative emotions requires having a solid repertoire of methods for expressing emotions.

Why is this important? Because effective expression of emotions supports a more balanced autonomic nervous system, healthier immune functioning, and improved physical health. Simply put, you reduce the likelihood of a pain flare when you recognize and express strong negative feelings such as anger, dread, or anxiety.

For example, picture yourself feeling angry at a friend for saying something unkind to you at a party. Imagine a continuum of possible levels of emotional expression. At one end of the continuum would be recognizing the feeling but otherwise doing or saying nothing. At the other end of the continuum would be confronting the friend directly and angrily about what she said. In between are several possible responses.

These options give you the flexibility to respond more appropriately to the unique details of the situation.

Here are some ways to express your emotions:

- **Talk to a different friend or confidant** about the incident and the feelings.

- **Walk and talk.** Getting up and moving your body can help to dislodge challenging and stuck feelings. Or go for a walk with a voice recorder so you can talk spontaneously on your stroll.

- **Write in a journal.** Notice that I list this both under the recognize and express sections here, as it can help with both functions. Ensure that you use short, simple phrases and include feeling words. Example: "When I heard you tell Frank at the party that I've been missing work so much lately, it made me feel angry and betrayed."

- **Write an unsent letter.** Since you will not be sending the letter, you can feel free and uninhibited to fully express the extent of all the embarrassment, hurt, and anger you might be feeling. This technique can also be used when you have strong negative emotions toward someone who is deceased.

- **Use the empty chair technique.** As a variation on the unsent letter, sit down and face an empty chair while imagining that the person you want to address is sitting in it. Then fully express your feelings toward the "person" in the empty chair. You will still get the benefits because you will have succeeded in the necessary steps of recognizing and then expressing the tough feelings.

- **Confront the person directly.** Sometimes nothing substitutes for talking directly to the person you feel bothered by. If you talk to the person you feel upset by, you might consider writing an unsent letter to crystallize your emotions before speaking to them.

CONCLUDING THOUGHTS ON THE TWO-STEP MODEL FOR RESOLVING DIFFICULT EMOTIONS

Remember that calm, clear identification and expression of your difficult emotions is more effective than yelling and accusations. That's why the pressure-cooker model is obsolete. Stay with the format of using "I feel" statements. Rather than saying, "You're so mean and thoughtless for what you said," it's far more effective to say, "I felt angry and hurt when you talked about my headaches with others like you did with Suzy." Keep in mind that resolution of difficult emotions can be achieved without necessarily talking directly to the person you're upset with.

These are just a few of many possible strategies for expressing and resolving negative emotions. Experiment with several of these methods and see which ones work best for you. Effective management of difficult emotions is one of the best medicines you can use for reducing pain flare-ups and improving your long-term health.

CHAPTER 25

Physical Exercise: What Kinds and How Much

Physical exercise is a powerful component of the ABC healing plan. Once you get going, you'll enjoy the benefits of regular physical exercise—the feelings of strength, energy, endurance, and hopefulness.

Inactivity leads to stiff muscles, decreased mobility, and decreased strength. These can all worsen the symptoms of chronic pain. Engaging in a regular exercise routine can help you manage your symptoms and improve your overall health. Exercise has been clearly demonstrated to be an effective and important treatment for all kinds of chronic pain. It can help to decrease inflammation, increase strength and mobility, improve mood, and decrease the intensity and intrusiveness of your pain.

What is exercise? Any activity that requires physical effort. It is used to improve fitness and health, in addition to reducing the symptoms of chronic pain.

Categories of exercise include aerobic (cardiovascular), strength training, and stretching.

- **Aerobic (Cardiovascular) Exercise:** Moderate–intensity physical activity that gradually increases your heart rate and breathing rate. This will help you to be more active for a longer period, with reduced pain. Examples include walking, biking, swimming, tai chi, tennis, and dancing. Even taking the stairs (rather than the elevator), parking a bit away from the store to walk a little farther, and doing housework count as aerobic exercise.

In particular, walking deserves special attention. The most powerful predictor of success in chronic pain rehabilitation is *daily distance walked,* according to many research studies as well as my years of clinical experience. It is not even necessary to walk particularly fast. Rather, what is most important is that you walk daily, gradually increasing the distance walked. You may start with as little as half a block, eventually working your way up to a mile or more.

- **Strength Training Exercise:** Building muscle strength and endurance will help you lessen your pain. This may include using weights, machines, kettle bells, stretch bands, or your body weight (such as doing push-ups or pull-ups).

- **Stretching Exercise:** Stretching is an essential part of the healing process. Healing from chronic pain requires muscles and connective tissue that are both strong and flexible. Stretching improves your mobility, encourages proper joint movement, and reduces pain.

HOW DOES EXERCISE REDUCE PAIN?

Exercise reduces pain and triggers self-healing resources in multiple ways. Exercise causes your brain and spinal cord to release natural painkilling hormones that turn off pain signals and calm your mood. Exercise also triggers your immune system to release natural hormones that heal injured tissues, reduce inflammation, and reduce pain signals. Physical activity improves the strength and overall health of muscle tissue, plus it prompts your muscles to release natural hormones that block pain signals from reaching your brain.

ADDITIONAL BENEFITS FROM EXERCISES FOR REDUCING CHRONIC PAIN

Physical activity also provides improvements in these areas:

- Energy
- Fatigue
- Strength
- Overall mood
- Physical fitness and function
- Depression
- Anxiety

- Sleep
- Body weight
- Blood pressure
- Glucose levels
- Resilience
- Quality of life

You and your healing team should establish the specific steps of your exercise plan. Keep in mind these general considerations about exercise (source: University of Iowa Healthcare Program):

THE GOAL IS TO BE MORE ACTIVE

For aerobic exercise, generally start with five to ten minutes daily, ultimately reaching a goal of thirty minutes or more each day. Keep your aerobic exercise at moderate intensity, ranging from 3 to 6 on a ten-point scale.

For strength training exercise, you can start with as little as one set of repetitions, ultimately building up to three sets of repetitions.

BE AWARE OF OBSTACLES TO REGULAR EXERCISE

Many patients with chronic pain may feel anxious about starting or continuing an exercise program. Common fears are that it will be uncomfortable and actually worsen their pain. Some are concerned that they don't have enough time to exercise regularly. Some are afraid that they don't know the correct way to do their exercises and will injure themselves.

While these concerns are common, please be reassured that physical exercise is a safe and effective healing strategy, especially when you establish an individualized exercise plan with your healing team.

SAFEGUARDS TO SUPPORT ONGOING REGULAR EXERCISE

Make a list of activities you would like to do if you were stronger and more fit. Examples might be: "I'd like to play golf twice a week," or "I'd like to attend my cousin's wedding without feeling exhausted." Make a list of likely excuses that might get in the way of regular exercise, such as "I'm too tired," "I'm too busy to take the time to exercise today," or "These exercises aren't going to make any difference in my pain anyway." Then come up with ways to respond if these excuses pop up. Tell a trusted friend when you start your exercise plan. Even better, plan to exercise with that friend or join a group exercise program.

KEEP IN CLOSE COMMUNICATION WITH YOUR HEALING TEAM

Note: As with all strategies discussed in the ABC plan, be sure to consult your physician and healing team before starting an individualized exercise program. Specific exercises may vary depending on the origin of your chronic pain. Certain conditions, such as fibromyalgia, may lead to increased pain with exercise, so start slow and monitor your symptoms.

Here are some common questions likely to emerge as you begin your plan:

- Which kinds of exercise are the best for my chronic pain?

- Is exercise safe?

- What should I do if my pain increases with exercise?

- Which medicines affect my ability to exercise?

- What are warning signs that I should stop exercising?

- What if I want to push longer or harder than the time/intensity limits I've adopted?

Your healing team will be able to provide individualized responses to your questions. Eventually you will hone in on an exercise regimen that works best for you.

CHAPTER 26

Eight Steps for Handling a Pain Flare

In my experience, one of the most difficult issues that any chronic pain patient struggles with is coping with a pain flare (otherwise referred to as a relapse, or setback). Everyone healing from chronic pain will encounter these occasional episodes periodically. Flares are not unexpected, but can be profoundly disruptive to your healing progress unless you are prepared with knowledge of flares as well as an effective plan for responding to one.

What follows here are specific suggestions for navigating this sometimes-tricky path, beginning with the story of Josh.

Josh, a forty-three-year-old father of two, had suffered from chronic low back pain for ten years following a work-related injury. He has been participating in the ABC method in the past year and was feeling hopeful due to making steady, incremental progress.

At one point he received an urgent call from a close friend who had to move out of his apartment on a deadline and needed help carrying a large chair from the living room. Feeling generally improved, Josh agreed to do it, eager to help. By the next day, Josh's back pain had increased drastically, causing heightened sharpness and tightness from his right hip, radiating down his right leg. Two weeks later, the pain had remained unchanged. He started to feel not only disappointed, but also increasingly angry. He became self-critical and told me, "If I just hadn't been so stupid in agreeing to move that chair!" The anger eventually morphed into hopelessness, and he feared that all the progress that he had previously made was now lost.

I explained to him that setbacks are common as part of the path to lasting healing, and that this didn't mean that his progress wouldn't continue.

As I discussed earlier in Chapter 10, "Your Healing Map," the notion of two steps forward and one step back is vital to understand when you are striving for permanent healing for your chronic pain. We humans seem to be hardwired to change in this type of pattern. It's almost as if once we make a new change, our body/mind system needs a little time to incorporate the change, and then reverts back a little bit to the old way of feeling before permanently moving forward.

Please remember that the changes that you make are not simply a matter of a different pain medication, a different exercise, a different thought, or a different nutritional supplement. The steps you are taking are changing your physiology. They are changing the cascades of neurotransmitters and hormones that influence the communication pathways between all the structures in your pain network. You are taking advantage of positive neuroplasticity, meaning that you are in the process of literally creating new, healthier neural pathways in your brain and nervous system. This takes time, and it more often follows an up and down trajectory, rather than a straight line to a pain-free life.

EIGHT STEPS FOR DEALING WITH PAIN FLARES AND TEMPORARY SETBACKS

In my previous book, *Trust Your Gut*, I described some time-tested strategies for effectively dealing with relapses of abdominal pain, and these steps are equally relevant for responding to flare episodes of all kinds of chronic pain.

1. Breathe. First, take a deep breath. And then a few more.

2. Recognize. Our old friend awareness once again. Acknowledge that a pain flare is actually occurring. Keep in mind that pain flares are

a normal part of the healing process. It is common for symptoms to get a little worse after a period of progress, and then improve again.

3. Accept. Once you recognize that you are having a flare episode, the next step is to accept it rather than fight it. Reactions of anger, panic, frustration, and despair are normal, but they can also agitate your sensitized nervous system, heightening the intensity of the pain even more. It is safe to be less afraid of the heightened feelings of aching, burning, stabbing pain, and fatigue that occur with this flare-up. Don't let them scare you. This doesn't mean that you've lost your progress. It is a temporary one step back.

4. Allow. Make room for whatever difficult emotions may surface. Allow the feeling, remembering that, "This is scary (or sad, or frustrating, or demoralizing), but it's a normal part of the healing process, and it will pass." This activates the important capacity for self-soothing of difficult emotions and sensations (refer back to Chapter 24 on "Resolving Difficult Emotions and Their Physical Effects" for useful reminders on how to do this).

5. Get support: Let the people who are close to you know about your ABC healing program and its steps. When a setback occurs, turn to them for support and encouragement.

6. Stay the course. Now more than ever. Get back to the fundamentals and self-care skills of your ABC program. Do Limbic Retraining to sit with the heightened sensations and reduce the agitation. It's particularly helpful during pain flares. Stick with the foods and nutrients that are part of your individualized plan for healing. Reduce whatever stresses may be flared up in any of the categories of stress you may be experiencing. Make sure that you are allowing enough time for sleep. Use your new skills for taking the sting out of any particularly difficult emotions that may be stirred up during this flare episode.

7. Use the flare episode to your advantage. Although a setback can be worrisome or frustrating, it also allows for the opportunity to

gather valuable new information to add to your ABC healing plan. You may become aware of some new and different stresses, physical movements, or activities that may worsen your pain in ways that you weren't as aware of before the flare. Also, when you practice your Limbic Retraining during the flare episode, you may become aware of a useful clue about something that may have contributed to the flare that you can avoid in the future.

8. Take heart: it will get better.

After getting reassurance and reminders about the steps of getting through a flare episode successfully, Josh calmed down and regained some of his confidence. Dr. Weisberg worked with responding to the symptoms of his pain flare. Starting with Limbic Retraining, he encouraged Josh to find the place in his right hip and leg where the sharpness and tightness were most troubling.

As he had learned to do previously, he imagined that he was going to pull up a chair and sit right next to the sharp, tight sensation exactly the way it is, without trying to change it in any way. Eventually, he was able to do this. After about three minutes, he reported that the sharpness had moved from his right hip to his central low back, and the intensity had reduced from an 8 to a 4. He stayed with the sensation for another ten minutes without trying to change it. After some time had passed, he was calmer. He said, "I still feel the discomfort, but it doesn't feel as heavy or ominous now. It changed just enough to remind me that all this will pass."

Josh also learned an important lesson from this flare episode. In his zeal to return to normal life, he agreed to help move a heavy chair without first checking in with his body to tell if he really felt up to it. "At first, it's depressing to think that I can't just do any physical lifting that I feel like, whenever I like. But then my common sense kicks in and I realize that I now just need to listen to how my body feels first, before returning to heavy lifting. That's an adjustment I'm willing to make to feel better!"

At the next appointment, Josh reported, "The pain intensity has reduced a little. I don't like pain flares any better than I used to, but I'm reassured that they're a normal part of the healing process. I won't be quite as scared or discouraged the next time a pain flare occurs."

As Josh learned, the more you utilize these strategies, the less you will be thrown off track by the ups and downs that are a normal part of the trajectory of healing from chronic pain.

CONCLUSION:

Maintain Your Gains Now and in the Future

The skills that you have learned from the ABC method in this book will enable you to rebalance your life and learn to trust your body/mind's inherent inner healing resources for reclaiming your life from chronic pain.

An important part of this skillset is the ability to maintain your balance in the coming months and years as you experience inevitable life cycles of change. My goal for you is to continually practice the skills you learn in the ABC program, so they become ingrained habits. I want to make sure that what you have been working so hard to achieve becomes a sustainable lifestyle change, rather than a temporary improvement.

We have all heard this story. Every New Year, about half of all Americans vow to either lose weight, stop smoking, exercise regularly, or make other behavioral changes. By February many are backsliding, and by the following December, most are back where they started. Why does this happen? It's usually not a matter of willpower or laziness. Rather, *life happens in the meantime!* Unforeseen financial pressures happen. A pain flare gets you off track. Close friends and other supporters leave town, or are otherwise preoccupied. Most people tend to resist change, so inertia sets in. And many pain sufferers tend to postpone practicing their skills as they start to feel better.

To counteract the natural inertia that fights change, I will present some support skills for your continued progress. These additional skills will help you to solidify your follow-through with the ABC program as a permanent lifestyle change.

PAY VERY CLOSE ATTENTION TO EVEN SMALL IMPROVEMENTS

There are various reasons why you might not notice small improvements in your pain. One reason is that so many people learn to disconnect from feeling discomfort, so they don't feel when the discomfort starts to decrease a little. When you don't want to accept anything less than "having the pain disappear," noticing that the intensity has reduced from a 5 to a 3 may not seem very encouraging.

And yet—paying attention to these small improvements is part of what reduces the hopelessness that often accompanies chronic pain! This information is vital because so many chronic pain sufferers go through long periods of time when their symptoms feel unchanged for what feels like months. This is why so many of my patients with chronic pain feel frustrated and hopeless by the time they get to me.

When you notice the pain has reduced from a 5 to a 3, this is a golden opportunity for you pay very close attention to it. This is your chance to ask important questions—yet another dimension of Awareness from the ABC model. Take this opportunity to expand your awareness of what healing is like.

Fill in the following questions in your ABC journal when the pain has improved even a little:

- When I'm feeling better, how has my emotional state changed?

- How have my thoughts changed?

- How has my feeling of hopefulness for the future changed?

- Is my motivation for practicing self-care any different now?

- Do I view myself as a person any differently now?

REWARD YOURSELF FOR SMALL IMPROVEMENTS ALONG THE WAY

Jonah suffered with chronic neck and shoulder pain. He committed to regular daily practice of the skills in the ABC program, including relaxation exercises, Limbic Retraining, physical exercise, and stress management. He acknowledged feeling better, but wasn't really sure exactly how much he had improved.

"It's hard to tell how my progress is going," Jonah complained. "It's almost like I'm swimming in the ocean—I'm moving along and swimming a long way, but it's hard to tell how far I've come because when I look for my bearings, all I can see is more and more water on the horizon."

Jonah's concerns are very common among pain sufferers. The healing process is a marathon, not a sprint, and sometimes day-to-day changes may be hard to recognize.

And when you don't notice these changes, it's easier for fatigue, cynicism, and hopelessness to kick in. This is why it's very important to both recognize and reward each forward step.

For example, if you are starting breathing exercises, start with small goals first. Perhaps aim for doing the Somatic Focus Breathing exercise twice daily for one week. Mark your progress daily in a journal. And then when you have met that goal, acknowledge this as important! And give yourself a small reward. Something that is enjoyable for you. Perhaps put some dollars aside for a short getaway. Go to a music or dance performance you enjoy. Psychological research tells us that these positive reinforcements provide encouragement for keeping up your practice, serve as a tangible reminder that you are making progress, and make it more likely that you will maintain these practices regularly.

KEEP PRACTICING

The more consistent your practice is, the easier it will be for new behaviors and skills to take hold. This is what best supports the development of positive neuroplasticity. For example, if you are practicing stretches for your neck and back, commit the same regular times every day for at least two weeks to do those stretches. Once you prioritize it by committing a time slot in your schedule, the learning cues like time of day and location are the same every time. It makes it far more likely that it will get done. Doing various practices at the same time and place also supports the development of new behavior, skills, and even neural connections. This will get easier with time, and the benefits for your healing and relief will grow as your practice becomes more of a part of your daily routine.

BUILD RESILIENCE

Resilience is the capacity to respond well in the face of adversity such as tragedy, threats, or significant sources of stress (including workplace or financial worries, serious health problems, family and relationship problems). Being resilient doesn't mean you never go through periods of feeling drained, depressed, or discouraged. The road to resilience often involves going through emotional distress initially. However, resilience is a common attribute—one that can be improved by anyone by learning new thoughts, behaviors, and ways of responding emotionally.

What do we know about resilient people? They tend to exhibit the following characteristics:

- They can make realistic plans and then carry these plans through

- They have skills for clear communication and problem-solving

- They have skills for identifying and managing strong feelings

- They have realistic confidence in their strengths and abilities

Practicing the skills and strategies in the ABC program will help you build resilience. In particular, the following skills and attitudes will help you increase your resilience:

- **Increase self-awareness.** Awareness is one of the cornerstones of the ABC approach. Resilient people are aware of their situation, their physical and emotional responses, and of people around them. Developing your "awareness muscles" (cognitive, somatic, emotional) will improve your resilience.

- **Accept occasional setbacks.** Setbacks occur regularly in everyone's healing journey. Accepting this leads you toward developing better coping skills over time. This will reduce the hypersensitivity of your nervous system that aggravates your chronic pain.

- **Develop optimal control in situations when it is possible for you to do something constructive.** This is important because we know that pain sufferers can experience benefit when they feel that there is something to be done that can help, no matter how small.

- **Establish strong social support**, which may include family, friends, coworkers, and even online support groups. This doesn't mean that you must continually hang out with large groups of people, if that doesn't fit your style. Rather, it means identifying what level of support feels optimal for you, and then taking action to seek that out.

- **Be open to professional help.** It builds resilience to know that, in addition to the help of friends and family, you can avail the help of psychologists who are specifically trained to deal with demanding, stressful situations.

- Finally, one last pointer to help you maintain your gains into the future: **Take a day off.** As I like to remind my patients in the ABC program, "Everything in moderation—including moderation!" You will feel less resistance to a change plan that is flexible. Every seven or eight days, take a day off from working on any of the ABC exercises if you'd like.

CLOSING THOUGHTS— AND NEW BEGINNINGS

We have reached the end of this book, but it is only the beginning of your journey for lifelong healing from chronic pain. By learning and applying the skills and tools gained in this book, you are now embarking on a path of dynamic self-care to ensure vibrant good health now and in the future.

In your personalized ABC program, you have taken several steps to empower yourself. You have gained awareness of your body, your emotions, your stresses, and your diet. You have learned to balance your posture, your nervous system, your diet, your work schedule, and your posture. You have started to cultivate your innate self-healing capacities through self-hypnosis, physical exercise, and dealing effectively with troubling emotions.

You have brought together your own healing team of trusted health professionals to rely on for guidance and "course correction" on the healing journey.

You've also learned to ensure ongoing progress by setting specific goals and intentions for enduring lifestyle change. As we discussed earlier in the "Cultivate" section, the greatest performers in sports and the arts know that their progress never stands still. Baseball superstars continue to work at batting practice. World-class pianists keep practicing their scales. The greatest professional ballet dancers stretch and practice their craft daily. No one is ever done in their quest for mastery—it's a continual practice. Whether it's setting consistent time for calming exercises, practicing self-hypnosis regularly, taking time for stretching, or making beneficial dietary changes, you now know the importance of setting small, tangible goals, and acknowledging and rewarding yourself for small steps of improvement. You now know that the trajectory of healing progress is usually "two steps forward, one step back," and have a plan for dealing with the inevitable occasional setback or flare episode.

Know that this book is not only a roadmap to healing—it is also a trusted guide that you can refer back to over and over, whenever you need a little refresher, a little reminder, or a little encouragement and reassurance. Know that countless patients have successfully navigated the path to healing from chronic pain using the ABC method, and you are on your way as well!

Remember: the reward in committing to ongoing practice of the ABC method is the profound hopefulness and satisfaction that comes from unleashing the most powerful medicine of all—your own innate self-healing resources.

Acknowledgments

This book project started in December of 2018. The journey of bringing this vision to reality and completion is an arduous one, filled with plenty of twists and turns, hills and valleys, and more than a few dead ends. The process is demanding and sometimes disorienting. A community of professionals and dear friends cheered me on and provided help, skills, encouragement, and at times a much-needed roadmap to my goal. I want to express my profound gratitude to them.

I am deeply appreciative of my professional colleagues who provided valuable insights and input to my manuscript. Their valuable feedback was crucial in informing and shaping the final product. They include Suzanne Candell, PhD; Alfred Clavel, MD; Kevin Harrington, PhD; and Issac Marsolek, MD.

My colleagues from the American Society of Clinical Hypnosis comprise a wonderfully unique and supportive group of professionals. They all work from an integrative medicine perspective, synthesizing multiple scientific perspectives. Our discussions over the years have benefited me greatly and have made me a better clinician. Special thanks to Elgan Baker, PhD; Thomas Barr, PhD; Carolyn Daitsch, PhD; Louis Damis, PhD; Sheryll Daniel, PhD; George Glaser, LCSW; Steven Gurgevich, PhD; Daniel Kohen, MD; Stephen Lankton, LCSW; Marc Oster, PsyD; Akira Otani, EdD; Maggie Phillips, PhD; Maryanna Polhukin, MD; David Reid, PsyD; Eric Spiegel, PhD; Lawrence Sugarman, MD; Eva Szigethy, PhD, MD; Judy Thomas, DDS; Linda Thompson, PhD; and David Wark, PhD.

This book was significantly influenced by my experiences over thirty-four years as a clinician and co-owner of the Minnesota Head and Neck Pain Clinic in St. Paul, Minnesota. My understanding of pain medicine and its treatment has been wonderfully enriched through my interactions

RESTORE YOUR LIFE FROM CHRONIC PAIN

with colleagues including Miles Belgrade, MD; Alfred Clavel, MD; Diane Clavel, NP; James Fricton, DDS, Subha Giri, DDS; Dennis Haley, DDS; Cory Herman, DDS; Emily Kahnert, DPT; Bonnie Penn, PT; and Eric Schiffman, DDS.

In particular, I am profoundly grateful for my friendship and professional collaboration with Alfred Clavel, MD. For over thirty years of treating patients and teaching together, we have been engaged in a wonderful, ongoing discussion about the nature of chronic pain and its treatment. He is a unique and gifted pain clinician, and I continue to benefit greatly from knowing him.

I am indebted to Steve LeBeau, my book editor. Steve possesses a unique gift for taking complex concepts from pain medicine and breaking them down into simpler, more accessible language. He provided frequent reminders of the importance of telling stories for bringing scientific principles to life. Just like my favorite professors from professional training days, he challenged me to take complicated terms from neuroscience literature and translate them into understandable ideas. He was the book editor for my previous book *Trust Your Gut*, and his skillful wordsmanship helped once again to bring my goal of a readable, accessible guide for patients and their families to fruition.

Dr. Marc Schoen has been a wonderfully steadfast and supportive friend for many years. As a clinical psychologist and published author, he understands the challenges of completing a book such as this and I appreciate his insights and care.

I want to acknowledge Publisher Brenda Knight, Managing Editor Robin Miller, and the rest of the great team at Mango Publishing. Brenda has consistently expressed great enthusiasm for this book project, convinced of its potential to help many people in pain. She and the rest of the team did an outstanding job of supporting and propelling the project along to completion.

Finally, I wish to acknowledge all the patients who arrived at our clinic and my practice feeling exhausted, exasperated, and hopeless. Years ago, such a patient showed up at my office. As we started working together, he said to me, "Dr Weisberg, when you talk about hope, I don't want you to just paste a smiley face over a pile of crap!" I wrote this book to share the message that there can be realistic hope, that life in fact *can* get better. For those who want to take control of their health, there are ways to get there. It is an honor and a privilege to participate in the lives and treatment of many, many patients who have journeyed the path from suffering to relief, from hopelessness to hope. With every passing year in clinical practice, I am humbled and inspired, consistently reminded of the miraculous self-healing capacities we all possess. My patients continue to be my greatest teachers. To all of them, a profound thank you.

About the Author

Mark B. Weisberg, PhD, ABPP, is a clinical health psychologist. He is a community adjunct professor in the Center for Spirituality and Healing at the University of Minnesota. He is a member of the American Academy of Pain Medicine and a fellow of the American Psychological Association and American Society of Clinical Hypnosis. For the last several years, he has been a co-owner of the Minnesota Head and Neck Pain Clinic, an integrative chronic pain clinic in the Twin Cities. He has been involved in clinical practice, teaching, and consultation in integrative medicine for the last thirty years. He is the bestselling author of *Trust Your Gut*, and resides in Minneapolis, Minnesota. Visit Dr. Weisberg at www. drmarkweisberg.com.

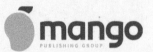

Mango Publishing, established in 2014, publishes an eclectic list of books by diverse authors—both new and established voices—on topics ranging from business, personal growth, women's empowerment, LGBTQ studies, health, and spirituality to history, popular culture, time management, decluttering, lifestyle, mental wellness, aging, and sustainable living. We were named 2019 *and* 2020's #1 fastest growing independent publisher by *Publishers Weekly*. Our success is driven by our main goal, which is to publish high quality books that will entertain readers as well as make a positive difference in their lives.

Our readers are our most important resource; we value your input, suggestions, and ideas. We'd love to hear from you—after all, we are publishing books for you!

Please stay in touch with us and follow us at:

Facebook: Mango Publishing

Twitter: @MangoPublishing

Instagram: @MangoPublishing

LinkedIn: Mango Publishing

Pinterest: Mango Publishing

Newsletter: mangopublishinggroup.com/newsletter

Join us on Mango's journey to reinvent publishing, one book at a time.

Printed in the USA
CPSIA information can be obtained
at www.ICGtesting.com
JSHW031748300524
64052JS00007B/12

9 781684 814220